IRRITABLE BOWEL SYNDROME

Irritable Bowel Syndrome

NEW IDEAS AND INSIGHTS INTO PATHOPHYSIOLOGY

Edited by N.W. Read

Professor of Gastrointestinal Physiology and Nutrition,
University of Sheffield

OXFORD

BLACKWELL SCIENTIFIC PUBLICATIONS

LONDON EDINBURGH BOSTON

MELBOURNE PARIS BERLIN VIENNA

© 1991 by
Blackwell Scientific Publications
Editorial Offices:
Osney Mead, Oxford OX2 0EL
25 John Street, London WC1N 2BL
23 Ainslie Place, Edinburgh EH3 6AJ
3 Cambridge Center, Cambridge
    Massachusetts 02142, USA
54 University Street, Carlton
    Victoria 3053, Australia

Other Editorial Offices:
Arnette SA
2, rue Casimir-Delavigne
75006 Paris
France

Blackwell Wissenschaft
Meinekestrasse 4
D-1000 Berlin 15
Germany

Blackwell MZV
Feldgasse 13
A-1238 Wien
Austria

First published 1991

Set by Excel Typesetters Company,
Hong Kong
Printed and bound in Great Britain by
Hartnolls Ltd, Bodmin, Cornwall

DISTRIBUTORS

Marston Book Services Ltd
PO Box 87
Oxford OX2 0DT
(*Orders*: Tel: 0865 791155
          Fax: 0865 791927
          Telex: 837515)
USA
  Mosby-Year Book, Inc.
  11830 Westline Industrial Drive
  St Louis, Missouri 63146
  (*Orders*: Tel: 800 633-6699)

Canada
  Mosby-Year Book, Inc.
  5240 Finch Avenue East
  Scarborough, Ontario
  (*Orders*: Tel: 416 298-1588)

Australia
  Blackwell Scientific Publications
  (Australia) Pty Ltd
  54 University Street
  Carlton, Victoria 3053
  (*Orders*: Tel: 03 347-0300)

British Library
Cataloguing in Publication Data

Irritable bowel syndrome.
  1. Man. Intestines. Irritable bowel
  syndrome
  I. Read, N.W.
  616.34

ISBN 0-632-02555-7

Contents

List of Contributors

P.L.R. Andrews BSc, PhD *Department of Physiology, St George's Hospital Medical School, Cranmer Terrace, Tooting, London SW17 0RE, UK*

J.R. Barton MB, BS, MRCP *University of Edinburgh Gastrointestinal Unit, Western General Hospital, Crewe Road South, Edinburgh EH4 2XU, UK*

F. Cervero MB, ChB, PhD *Director Visceral Sensation Research Group, Department of Physiology, University of Bristol Medical School, University Walk, Bristol BS8 1TD, UK*

S.M. Collins MB, BS, FRCP(UK), FRCPC *Director Intestinal Diseases Research Unit, McMaster University, Hamilton, Ontario, Canada*

A.W. Cuthbert BSc, MA, PhD, FRS *Department of Pharmacology, University of Cambridge, Tennis Court Road, Cambridge CB2 1QJ, UK*

D. Grundy BSc, PhD *Department of Biomedical Science, University of Sheffield, Sheffield S10 2TN, UK*

P.H. Howarth BSc, DM, MRCP *Centre Block, Southampton General Hospital, Southampton SO9 4XY, UK*

J.O. Hunter MA, MD, FRCP *Addenbrooke's Hospital, Hills Road, Cambridge CB2 2QQ, UK*

P.B. Miner Jr MD *University of Kansas Medical Center, Kansas City, Kansas, USA*

N.W. Read MD, FRCP *Centre for Human Nutrition, Northern General Hospital, Herries Road, Sheffield S5 7AU, UK*

H.L. Smart DM, MRCP *Broadgreen Hospital, NHS Trust, Thomas Drive, Liverpool LI4 3LB, UK*

V. Stanghellini MD *1st Medical Clinic, University di Bologna, Ospedales Orsola, Via Massarentia, I-40138 Bologna, Italy*

D.G. Thompson MD, MRCP *Hope Hospital, University of Manchester School of Medicine, Eccles Old Road, Salford M6 3HD, UK*

P.J. Whorwell BSc, MD, FRCP *University Hospital of South Manchester, Nell Lane, West Didsbury, Manchester M20 8LR, UK*

D.L. Wingate DM, FRCP *Department of Gastrointestinal Science, London Hospital Medical College, Turner Street, London E1 2AD, UK*

Preface

The functional bowel complaints, including irritable bowel syndrome, are perhaps the commonest cause of referral to a gastroenterologist, yet these conditions are very poorly understood. This book focuses on some of the recent developments that are relevant to our understanding of functional bowel disorders. These include insights into the operation of the enteric nervous system, the interface between the autonomic nerves in the gut, gastrointestinal sensitivity, the immunology of the gut and the linkage between the immune system and nervous reflexes. The aim of the book is to stimulate thought and research into functional bowel disorders by examining them from new perspectives.

N.W. Read

Section 1
Introduction

1 *The Neurotic Bowel: A Paradigm for the Irritable Bowel Syndrome*

N.W. Read

WHAT IS THE IRRITABLE BOWEL SYNDROME?

This is a subject on which no two investigators agree. The safest definition is the broadest; the irritable bowel syndrome (IBS) is the association of abdominal discomfort with an alteration in bowel habit for which no cause can be found on routine clinical investigation. The alteration in bowel habit may be diarrhoea or constipation, or erratic defaecation consisting of alternating diarrhoea and constipation. Irritable bowel syndrome also encompasses a variety of other gastrointestinal symptoms (Table 1.1), but patients frequently complain of symptoms referable to organs outside the gastrointestinal tract (see Chapter 5). The broader the definition, the less we understand.

In recent years, there has been a tendency to restrict the definition (Thompson *et al.*, 1989). Thus, patients with large volume watery diarrhoea, and patients with chronic persistent abdominal pain that is not associated with any change in bowel habit, would not be regarded as having IBS. Patients with severe constipation who have slow transit times and defaecate less than twice a week may also be excluded.

ONE DISEASE OR SEVERAL?

Most clinical investigators who have studied IBS would, I think, agree that it consists of different pathophysiological subsets and effective therapy can only result from the accurate identification of these subsets.

The most useful method to establish subsets must be from their response to specific therapy. Thus there is a cohort of IBS patients whose symptoms disappear when they abolish milk from the diet. There is another group whose symptoms remit when they take bile acid binding agents such as cholestyramine. Such observations have established 'lactose intolerance' (Newcomer & McGill, 1983; Eastwood *et al.*, 1984) and 'bile acid malabsorption' (Thaysen & Pedersen, 1976; Merrick *et al.*, 1985) as subsets of IBS, but patients

Table 1.1. Symptoms frequently reported by patients with IBS

Bloating
Early satiety
Nausea
Heartburn
Feeling of incomplete evacuation
Borborygmi
Flatulence
Urgency
Passage of mucus
Abdominal pain, relieved by defaecation
Abdominal distension
Frequent desire to defaecate
Alternating bowel habit

with these conditions form a very small percentage of the the total number of patients with IBS. For most patients, there is currently no effective or specific treatment for IBS, although some are helped by symptomatic therapy with antispasmodics, antidiarrhoeal agents (Cann *et al.*, 1984b) or adjusting the intake of dietary fibre (Cann *et al.*, 1984a).

Classification by symptoms

There is a general feeling that it should be possible to categorize patients on the basis of their presenting symptoms. I suspect that if this were feasible, it would have been done a long time ago. The classical symptoms of IBS—feeling of incomplete evacuation, abdominal discomfort relieved by defaecation, bloating after meals and passage of rectal mucus—are non-specific (Manning *et al.*, 1978). The same symptoms can be found in other colonic diseases such as ulcerative colitis (Rao *et al.*, 1988a) and solitary rectal ulcer syndrome (Sun *et al.*, 1989). They can be induced in normal volunteers, who have been made constipated by ingestion of an opiate-like antidiarrhoeal agent (Oettle & Heaton, 1987). Since the afferent nerve supply to the rectum is more dense than in other regions of the colon, these symptoms probably give no more information than indicating that something is wrong with the rectum.

Bowel habit

In many studies, patients with IBS have been segregated on the basis of their predominant bowel habit. After all, it seems obvious, for example, that patients who present predominantly with diarrhoea should have a different disease mechanism than those who have constipation. This distinction may be justified on therapeutic grounds inasmuch as diarrhoea can be treated symptomatically with small doses of opiate-like antidiarrhoeal agents such as loperamide (Cann *et al.*, 1984b). This contrasts with the symptoms of constipation which may respond to bulk laxatives or increasing the dietary intake of fibre (Cann *et al.*, 1984a). Unfortunately symptomatic treatment is no cure and, while it may be useful for the target symptom, it may make other symptoms worse. For example, the treatment of constipation with an increased dietary intake of bran. Bran is an effective treatment for constipation in IBS patients (Cann *et al.*, 1984a). However, it may exacerbate symptoms of pain, distension and flatulence.

Symptomatic treatment cannot be used as a basis for classification unless it is directed at the pathophysiological mechanism. So is there any data to suggest that IBS patients with diarrhoea have a different disease than patients with constipation? Cann has shown that small bowel and whole gut transit times are longer in patients with constipation than in patients with diarrhoea (Cann *et al.*, 1983), but the considerable overlap between the groups and the observations that nearly all the values fall within the normal range does not support segregation on the basis of bowel habit. Kellow and his colleagues have shown similar abnormalities in small bowel motor activity irrespective of their predominant bowel habit (Kellow *et al.*, 1990). Studies on colonic motor activity have reported differences between patients with diarrhoea and those with constipation (Chaudhary & Truelove, 1961; Connell, 1962; Whitehead *et al.*, 1980), but many IBS patients fall into a middle ground where the distinction between diarrhoea and constipation is blurred and the presentation may change from day to day and even within the same day. Finally, although enhanced rectal sensitivity is more common in IBS patients with diarrhoea (Prior *et al.*, 1990a), it can also be found in one-third of patients presenting with constipation (Prior *et al.*, 1990b). Thus, considering all the available data, I no longer feel that bowel habit is a useful criterion for the subdivision of IBS.

Not all patients, of course, have a predominant disturbance in bowel habit. A significant group have alternating diarrhoea and constipation. Both constipation and diarrhoea are terms that encompass a number of different presentations and a variety of pathophysiologies. The patient who passes frequent small faecal pellets probably has a different disease from the patient who passes a large volume of fluid stools once a day, although both complain of diarrhoea. The patient who only feels a desire to defaecate once a week almost certainly has a different disease than the patient who strains to squeeze out a faecal pellet five times a day, although both complain of constipation.

Tests of rectal sensitivity

I suspect that the best operative means of subdividing patients with IBS is by the use of physiological tests, but which test is the most relevant? Measurement of rectal sensitivity to balloon distension would be my first choice on the grounds that most IBS symptoms are based on rectal sensations.

Alison Prior and I have recently tested the sensitivity of the rectum to balloon distension in 55 patients with IBS (Prior *et al.*, 1990b). Thirty-two patients (58%) showed evidence of abnormal sensitivity in that they perceived a desire to defaecate and other sensations such as wind and pain at abnormally low volumes, while the remainder had normal rectal sensitivity. The patients in the sensitive group had abnormally reduced rectal compliance and they generated rectal contractions and internal sphincter relaxations at abnormally low rectal volumes. The IBS patients who did not have a sensitive rectum had normal values for rectal compliance and motor 'reactivity'. It is unlikely that the 'tighter' rectum causes the increased rectal sensitivity. Rectal compliance can be reduced in normal subjects by increasing the rate of ramp distension, but sensitivity is not enhanced under those circumstances; it is reduced (Sun *et al.*, 1990a). These observations suggest that the increased tonic and phasic rectal motor activity could be the result of rectal sensitization instead of the cause of it.

Do patients with the sensitive rectum present with different symptoms compared with the remainder of patients with IBS? The only symptom that is more common in patients with enhanced rectal sensitivity is a more frequent desire to defaecate (Prior *et al.*, 1990b). Other symptoms, such as abdominal pain relieved by defaecation and a feeling of incomplete evacuation, are found with equal frequency in the sensitive and non-sensitive groups.

Although a sensitive rectum was found in a high proportion of patients who presented with diarrhoea, it was not confined to that group. One-third of the patients, who complained of constipation, also had a 'sensitive rectum'; all of them had a frequent desire to defaecate, but they had to strain to pass small faecal pellets. A few years ago, we showed that hard objects are much more difficult to evacuate from the rectum when their diameter is reduced (Bannister *et al.*, 1987). Thus, I suspect that some IBS patients who complain of constipation have a rectum that is so sensitive they can perceive the entry of faecal pellets that would not cause any sensation in a normal subject. This produces a frequent desire to defaecate, but because the pellets are so small, they cannot be readily expelled without a great deal of effort. This may be why the patients with a sensitive rectum complain of constipation. Tests of rectal sensitivity distinguish these patients from the remainder of constipated patients who do not present with a frequent desire to defaecate.

Another striking association was that anxiety was much more common in patients with the sensitive rectum (Prior *et al.*, 1990b). This is interesting because Erkenbrecht (1989) recently showed that experimental stress can increase the sensitivity of the rectum.

The phenomenon of rectal sensitization might be called the neurotic bowel. This term is operational, but focuses attention on the enteric nervous system (ENS) and also on the possible importance of psychological mechanisms. The implication of this terminology is that like the neurotic person, the neurotic bowel is also hypersensitive and hyperreactive to stimuli. Hypersensitivity and hyperreactivity may not necessarily be confined to the rectum. Previous studies in IBS have shown that the oesophagus (Edwards, 1974; Richter *et al.*, 1986), the small intestine (Moriarty & Dawson, 1982) and the colon (Ritchie, 1973; Swarbrick *et al.*, 1980) can also show increased sensitivity to balloon distension, but nobody knows whether IBS patients who have a tender oesophagus, for example, necessarily have a sensitive rectum.

Furthermore balloon distension is not the only stimulus to which the gut may be sensitive or hyperreactive. Studies have shown an increased reactivity of the rectosigmoid colon (Connell *et al.*, 1965; Kock *et al.*, 1968; Sun *et al.*, 1990b) and the ileum (Kellow & Phillips, 1987) to a meal or infusions of cholecystokinin (Harvey & Read, 1973; Kellow *et al.*, 1988) or bile acids (Taylor *et al.*, 1980) in some patients with IBS. Bond and Levitt showed that some patients with functional bowel disorders exhibited more symptoms in response to intestinal infusion of an inert gas (Lasser *et al.*, 1975), while Cann and his colleagues showed that patients with IBS had more symptoms after ingestion of a test meal containing baked beans, especially when the meal reached the colon and produced gas (Cann *et al.*, 1983). It is not known whether patients who show increased rectosigmoid responses to distension are also those who show increased responses to chemical stimuli.

Finally, recent studies have demonstrated a high incidence of urodynamic abnormalities (Whorwell *et al.*, 1986), such as detrusor instability, and bronchial hyperreactivity (White *et al.*, 1988) in patients with IBS. Taken collectively, these studies suggest that the whole gastrointestinal tract and perhaps even the whole body may be abnormally sensitive in some patients with IBS, but this possibility can only be established when sensitivity or reactivity in different anatomical regions are tested in the same patient.

Adaptations for clearance

The changes in gastrointestinal motor activity, which have been described in some patients with IBS, suggest an adaptation for clearance of gut contents. The hypersensitive and hyperreactive rectum may be part of a mechanism for clearing the distal colon. An abnormal preponderance of clusters of contractions in the small intestine is said to be typical of IBS (Kellow & Phillips, 1987) (see

Chapter 3). Such clusters are thought to propel intestinal contents and can be associated with a rapid intestinal transit (Read, 1986). Another highly propulsive mode of small intestinal motor activity is the giant migrating contraction, which is also said to be more common in patients with IBS (Kellow & Phillips, 1987) and associated with pain. Recordings of myoelectrical activity in the colon of IBS patients with diarrhoea have demonstrated a preponderance of propagative spike bursts (Bueno *et al.*, 1980; Frexinos *et al.*, 1987). Intestinal transit times tend to be rapid in IBS patients with diarrhoea, most of whom have a sensitive rectum.

Clearance of the gut involves a change in motor activity and a stimulation of secretion. Factors that cause diarrhoea, such as chemicals, bacterial infections, neurotransmitters, induce both propagation and secretion (Read, 1986). Is there any evidence that the intestinal epithelium has adopted a secretory mode in patients with IBS? Excessive secretion of mucus is a feature of IBS. One type of IBS used to be called 'mucous colitis'. The only firmly documented evidence for hypersecretion in IBS can be found in a paper by Oddson *et al.* (1978), who demonstrated an enhanced secretory response to bile acids in the small intestine of patients with IBS.

Only the middle and the lower gastrointestinal tract are cleared by diarrhoea. The stomach and upper small intestine can be cleared by vomiting. Thus the high prevalence of upper gastrointestinal symptoms such as nausea and early satiety and the delays in gastric emptying that have been demonstrated in some patients with IBS (Cann *et al.*, 1983) may be an adaptation for clearance of the upper gut. Has the neurotic gut adopted the posture for clearance by vomiting as well as diarrhoea? The observations that have been carried out do not entirely support that hypothesis. Upper gastrointestinal symptoms are no more common in IBS patients with the 'sensitive rectum' than in patients who do not show rectal sensitivity (Prior *et al.*, 1990b), and delays in gastric emptying are frequently seen in patients who present with constipation (Cann *et al.*, 1983), most of whom do not exhibit rectal sensitivity.

What are the mechanisms of rectal sensitization?

The hyperreactive state of the bowel in IBS is reminiscent of other diseases, such as asthma. Bronchial hyperreactivity can, however, be the end result of a number of different pathophysiological mechanisms; inflammatory, allergic, psychogenic, irritation by dust or chemicals (see Chapter 16). It therefore seems unlikely that the hypersensitive and hyperreactive bowel can result from one single mechanism; the evidence suggests that, like asthma, this type of IBS represents a stereotyped response to a number of different sensitizing factors; chemical, physical, inflammatory or psychogenic.

It may be possible to gain insight into the mechanism responsible for sensitization by careful evaluation of symptoms and physiological tests. For example, those patients who exhibit sensitivity of the rectum may have a local cause such as colitis (Rao *et al.*, 1987), solitary rectal ulcer syndrome (Sun *et al.*, 1989) or malabsorption of bile acids (Edwards *et al.*, 1989). Those subjects, whose sensitivity extends to the upper gut but is not found in organs outside the gastrointestinal tract, could perhaps have an immunological mechanism associated with food intolerance (see Section 4) or an inflammatory condition involving several regions of the gut. Finally, sensitivity and hyperreactivity of several organs both within and outside the gut would perhaps be more in keeping with a psychological mechanism causing autonomic arousal.

Autonomic arousal

Several studies have shown that IBS patients have higher anxiety scores (Esler & Gouldston, 1973; Liss *et al.*, 1973; Young *et al.*, 1976; Whitehead *et al.*, 1980; Prior *et al.*, 1990b) and suffer more life stresses (Craig & Brown, 1984; Ford *et al.*, 1987) than the normal population, although some have suggested this may be one facet of self-selection by more neurotic individuals. Only those IBS patients with a high degree of neuroticism attend physicians (Whitehead *et al.*, 1988). Acute experimental stress can enhance the motor activity of the gut and cause pain (Almy & Toolin, 1947; Narducci *et al.*, 1985; Welgan *et al.*, 1988), and many IBS patients report that acute psychological stress is associated with onset or exacerbation of symptoms (Chaudhary & Truelove, 1962; Hislop, 1971). Exposure of human volunteers to mental stress can also increase the sensitivity of the rectum (Erkenbrecht, personal communication). Increased activity in the autonomic nerves is thought to modulate afferent transmission and visceral reflexes through a number of possible mechanisms (Mayer & Raybauld, 1989) (see Section 3).

Although it is tempting to link the effects of acute experimental stress to the characteristics of IBS, the type of stress that can be produced in the laboratory may be completely unlike the stresses that patients suffer from.

1 The nature of the stress may be quite different. The type of stress that 'upsets' people is often emotional stress of a highly personalized nature that cannot be mimicked in the laboratory.

2 The effects of acute predictable stress may be quite different from the chronic stresses that many patients are exposed to. Recently when rats were exposed to prolonged heavy metal music it was found that after several days the responses of strips of longitudinal muscle nerve to physical and chemical stimuli were markedly enhanced (see Chapter 14).

3 It is possible that the 'harmful' effects of stress are not so much caused by the positive effects of 'coping' with threat, but are due more to decompensation or exhaustion. Few studies have addressed this possibility.

In contrast to the physiological explanation for increased sensitivity, Latimer has suggested that patients with IBS may mislabel normal sensations as pain because of their high level of neuroticism (Latimer, 1981). This hypothesis would lead to the prediction that IBS patients would have lower pain thresholds for all types of bursts of stimuli. This is clearly not true, since Cook and his colleagues have recently shown that somatic pain thresholds in patients with IBS are in fact higher than they are in normal subjects (Latimer, 1981; Cook *et al.*, 1987).

Inflammation

The inflamed bowel is also hypersensitive and hyperreactive. Studies carried out recently in patients with ulcerative colitis showed that in the presence of active inflammation, patients exhibited all the symptoms of the irritable rectum; urgency, a frequent desire to defaecate, pain relieved by defaecation and feelings of incomplete evacuation (Rao *et al.*, 1988a). Moreover, distension of the rectum produced a desire to defaecate, and also pain volumes similar to those that evoked the same symptoms in patients with IBS but much lower than the volumes required in normal subjects (Rao *et al.*, 1987). As in IBS patients, the rectum and distal colon in patients with active colitis show a greater motor reactivity to distension and to infusion of large volumes of saline (Rao *et al.*, 1988b). This abnormal reactivity and sensitivity was not present in patients with quiescent colitis.

Similar hypersensitivity and hyperreactivity have been described in patients with the solitary rectal ulcer syndrome (Sun *et al.*, 1989) and also after infusion of relatively small (1–3 mmol/litre) concentrations of deoxycholic acid into the rectum of normal volunteers (Edwards *et al.*, 1989). Deoxycholic acid can cause mild inflammation of the colon and induce colonic secretion and propulsive motor activity (Binder, 1980; Snape *et al.*, 1980).

Inflammation results in a marked increase in afferent discharge in response to stimuli, and may make sensory receptors that are normally only responsive to high levels of stimulation respond to much lower levels (see Chapter 9), so that small degrees of distension or even normal contractile activity may be perceived as painful. It is not exactly certain how these changes can be brought about, but it is likely that the release of inflammatory mediators, such as prostanoids, bradykinins, serotonin and histamine from damaged tissues and from mast cells could modulate afferent discharge (see Chapter 14).

Sensitization by an immunological mechanism

There is a group of IBS patients whose symptoms commence with an attack of gastroenteritis on holiday (Chaudhary & Truelove, 1962). It is possible that this injury to the gut may have altered the permeability of the epithelium, allowing access of food antigens to immunoreactive cells in the submucosa. The gut of experimental animals can be sensitized to antigens by exposure during epithelial damage caused by parasitic infestation, or administration of bile acids, or even exposure to ultraviolet light (see Chapter 13). Repeated exposure to the antigen will cause a marked hypersecretion, an increase in motor activity, and a proliferation of mast cells (see Chapter 15).

The degranulation of mast cells is a powerful stimulus for the proliferation of more mast cells and also for the growth of nerves, which then interact with the mast cells. Recent experiments from Bienenstock's group (1987) have shown that it is possible to condition mast cell degranulation to a coadministered auditory stimulus. This interesting experiment could be directly relevant to IBS. Suppose, for example, the bowel became sensitized during an attack of gastroenteritis to common food antigens. After a time, this response to a specific food-associated stimulus could be conditioned into a non-specific response to the ingestion of food. This may explain the extreme difficulty of treating patients who claim to be upset by eating any food.

If mast cell degranulation was an important mediator of the symptoms of IBS, these should respond to specific mast cell stabilizers or antihistamines. To my knowledge there have been no formal studies on the effects of these agents on IBS, but anecdotal reports suggest they can be remarkably effective in some patients (see Chapter 15).

Therapeutic implications

Categorization of patients with IBS is only useful if it identifies groups that respond to specific and relevant therapies. Is there a method for desensitizing the rectum other than avoidance of stress or dietary regulation? Recently, new specific serotonin antagonists that are thought to block the 5-hydroxytryptamine (5HT$_3$) receptors on afferent nerves have been introduced. Preliminary results show that these agents reduce rectal sensitivity in IBS patients with the sensitive rectum and also reduce motor responses to ingestion of a fatty meal. These encouraging results should prompt therapeutic trials of these agents in IBS (Prior & Read, 1990).

PATIENTS WITH THE NON-SENSITIVE RECTUM

Little is known about the pathophysiological mechanisms in IBS patients who do not show physiological evidence of hypersensitivity or hyperreactivity. Many of them have a tendency to constipation. Severe slow transit constipation is not usually included as part of the spectrum of IBS, but it could represent the far end of the same disease. Many suspect that an important subset of patients with IBS have a neuropathy involving the enteric or autonomic nervous system (ANS) (see Chapter 3). Manometric studies have revealed bizarre small intestinal motor patterns, indicative of intestinal pseudo-obstruction in some patients whose presentation resembles a severe IBS (Stanghellini *et al.*, 1987). These abnormal patterns include failure to convert fasted to fed motor activity, impaired configuration and propagation of phase III of the migrating motor complex and prolonged non-propagative tonic and phasic activity (see Chapter 4). Neuropathic damage to the enteric and autonomic nerves is well described in diabetes mellitus, and it is possible that this condition could provide a model for understanding how disturbances in nervous control can affect gut function and symptoms.

Some patients, particularly those with bloating, flatulence and diarrhoea may have excessive carbohydrate fermentation. These symptoms can be reproduced in normal subjects by drinking large quantities of lactulose. The symptoms may be caused by excessive intake of fibre-rich foods, or particular sugars or sugar alcohols (Rumessen & Goodman-Hayer, 1988) or by a relative malabsorption of carbohydrate. People with lactase deficiency may have similar symptoms. Hunter's group have described a series of patients with 'functional' diarrhoea who respond to a diet that carefully excludes certain carbohydrate foods, in particular wheat flour (Alun-Jones *et al.*, 1982). The presence of gluten in wheat flour seems to impair the absorption of starch (Anderson *et al.*, 1981). When the starch gets into the large intestine, it is fermented to short chain fatty acids and gas, causing symptoms.

REFERENCES

Almy, T.P. & Toolin, M.N. (1947) Alterations in colonic function in man and distress. I. Experimental production of changes simulating the irritable colon. *Gastroenterology* 8, 616–626.

Alun-Jones, V.A., McLaughlan, P., Shorthouse, M. & Hunter, J. (1982) Food intolerance: a major factor in the pathogenesis of irritable bowel syndrome. *Lancet* ii, 1115–1117.

Anderson, I.H., Levin, A.S. & Levitt, M.D. (1981) Incomplete absorption of the carbohydrate in all-purpose wheat flour. *New Engl J Med* 304, 891–892.

Bannister, J.J., Dawson, P., Timms, J.M., Gibbons, C.G. & Read, N.W. (1987) Effect of the stool size and consistency on defaecation. *Gut* 28, 1246–1250.

Bienenstock, J., Perdue, M., Stanisz, A. *et al.* (1987) Neurohumoral regulation of gastrointestinal immunity. Editorial. *Gastroenterology* 93, 1431–1434.

Binder, H.J. (1980) Pathophysiology of bile acid and fatty acid induce diarrhoea. In Field, M., Fordtran, J.S. & Schultz, S.G. (eds), *Secretory Diarrhoea*, pp. 159–178. American Physiological Society, Bethesda, Maryland.

Bueno, L., Fioramonti, J., Ruckebusch, Y., Freckinos, J. & Coulom, P. (1980) Evaluation of colonic myoelectrical activity in health and functional disorders. *Gut* 21, 480–485.

Cann, P.A., Read, N.W., Brown, C., Hobson, N. & Holdsworth, C.D. (1983) The irritable bowel syndrome (IBS). Relationship of disorders in the transit of a single solid meal; the symptom patterns. *Gut* 24, 405–411.

Cann, P.A., Read, N.W. & Holdsworth, C.D. (1984a) What is the benefit of coarse wheat bran in patients with the irritable bowel syndrome? *Gut* 25, 168–173.

Cann, P.A., Read, N.W., Holdsworth, C.D. & Barends, D. (1984b) The role of loperamide and placebo in the management of the irritable bowel syndrome (IBS). *Dig Dis Sci* 29, 239–247.

Chaudhary, N.A. & Truelove, S.C. (1961) Human colonic motility— a comparative study of normal subjects and patients with ulcerative colitis and patients with the irritable bowel syndrome. 1. Resting patterns. *Gastroenterology* 40, 1–17.

Chaudhary, N.A. & Truelove, S.C. (1962) The irritable colon syndrome. A study of the clinical features, predisposing causes and prognosis in 130 cases. *Q J Med* 31, 307–323.

Connell, A.M. (1962) The motility of the pelvic colon. Part II. Paradoxical motility in diarrhoea and constipation. *Gut* 3, 342–348.

Connell, A.M., Jones, F.A. & Rowlands, E.N. (1965) Motility of the pelvic colon; pain associated with colonic hypermotility after meals. *Gut* 6, 105–112.

Cook, I.J., Vandeen, A. & Collins, S.M. (1987) Patients with irritable bowel syndrome have greater pain tolerance than normal subjects. *Gastroenterology* 93, 727–733.

Craig, T.K.J. & Brown, G.W. (1984) Goal frustration and life events in the aetiology of painful gastrointestinal disorders. *J Psychosom Res* 28, 411–421.

Eastwood, M.A., Walton, B.A. & Brydon, W.G. (1984) Faecal weight constitutents, colonic motility and lactose tolerance in the irritable bowel syndrome. *Digestion* 390, 7–12.

Edwards, C.A., Baxter, J., Brown, S., Bannister, J.J. & Read, N.W. (1989) Effect of bile acids on anorectal function in humans. *Gut* 30, 383–386.

Edwards, D.A.W. (1974) In Vantrappen, G. & Hellemans, J. (eds) *Handbook Der Inneren Medizin*, pp. 112–124, Springer-Verlag, Berlin.

Erkenbrecht, J.F. (1989) Noise and intestinal motor alterations. In Bueno, L., Collins, S. & Junien, J.L. (eds), *Stress and Digestive Motility*. John Libby, Paris.

Esler, M.D. & Gouldston, K.J. (1973) Levels of anxiety and colonic disorders. *New Engl J Med* 288, 16–20.

Ford, M.J., Millar, P.M., Eastwood, J. & Eastwood, M.A. (1987) Life events, psychiatric illness and the irritable bowel syndrome. *Gut* 28, 160–165.

Frexinos, J., Fioramonti, J. & Bueno, L. (1987) Colonic myoelectrical activity in IBS painless diarrhoea. *Gut* 28, 1613–1618.

Harvey, R.F. & Read, A.E. (1973) Effect of cholecystokinin on colonic motility and symptoms in patients with the irritable bowel syndrome. *Lancet* i, 1–3.

Hislop, I.G. (1971) Psychological significance of the irritable colon syndrome. *Gut* 12, 452–457.

Kellow, J.E. & Phillips, S.F. (1987) Altered small bowel motility in irritable bowel syndrome is correlated with symptoms. *Gastroenterology* 92, 1885–1893.

Kellow, J.E., Miller, L.J., Phillips, S.F. *et al.* (1988) Dysmotility of the small intestine is provoked by stimuli in the irritable bowel syndrome. *Gut* 29, 1236–1243.

Kellow, J.E., Gill, R.C. & Wingate, D.L. (1990) Prolonged ambulant recordings of small bowel motility demonstrate abnormalities in the irritable bowel syndrome. *Gastroenterology* **98**, 1208–1218.

Kock, N.J., Hulten, N.L. & Leandoer, L. (1968) A study of the motility in different parts of the human colon. Resting activity, response to feeding and to prostigmine. *Scand J Gastroenterol* **3**, 163–169.

Lasser, R.B., Bond, J.H. & Levitt, M.D. (1975) The role of intestinal gas in functional abdominal pain. *New Engl J Med* **293**, 524–526.

Latimer, P.R. (1981) Irritable bowel syndrome: a behaviour model. *Behav Res Ther* **19**, 475–483.

Liss, J.L., Alpers, D., Woodruff, R.A. (1973) The irritable colon syndrome and psychiatric illness. *Dis Nervous System* **34**, 151–157.

Manning, P.T., Thompson, W.G. & Heaton, K.W. (1978) Towards positive diagnosis of the irritable bowel. *Br Med J* **2**, 653–654.

Mayer, E.A. & Raybauld, H. (1989) The role of neural control in GI motility and visceral pain. In Snape, W.J. (ed), *Pathogenesis of Functional Bile Disease. Topics in Gastroenterology*, pp. 13–35. Plenum, London.

Merrick, M.V., Eastwood, M.A. & Ford, M.J. (1985) Is bile acid malabsorption under-diagnosed? An evaluation of diagnosis by measurement of SEHCAT retention. *Br Med J* **290**, 665–668.

Moriarty, K.J. & Dawson, A.M. (1982) Functional abdominal pain: further evidence that the whole gut is affected. *Br Med J* **284**, 1670–1672.

Narducci, F., Snape, W.J. & Battle, W.M. (1985) Increased colonic motility during exposure to a stressful situation. *Dig Dis Sic* **30**, 40–44.

Newcomer, A.D. & McGill, D.B. (1983) Irritable bowel syndrome. Role of lactose deficiency. *Mayo Clin Proc* **58**, 339–341.

Oddson, E., Rask-Madsen, J. & Krag, E. (1978) A secretory epithelium of the small intestine with increased sensitivity to bile acids in irritable bowel syndrome associated with diarrhoea. *Scand J Gastroenterol* **13**, 409–416.

Oettle, G.J. & Heaton, K.W. (1987) Is there a relationship between symptoms of the irritable bowel syndrome and objective measurements of large bowel function? A longitudinal study. *Gut* **28**, 146–149.

Prior, A. & Read, N.W. (1990) Reduction of rectal sensitivity and postprandial motility by granisetron, a $5HT_3$ receptor antagonist in patients with irritable bowel syndrome. *Gut* **31**, A1174.

Prior, A., Maxton, D.G. & Whorwell, P.J. (1990a) Anorectal manometry in the irritable bowel syndrome. Differences between diarrhoea- and constipation-predominant subjects. *Gut* **31**, 458–462.

Prior, A., Sorial, E., Sun, W.M. & Read, N.W. (1990b) Rectal sensitivity—a rational means of categorizing patients in the irritable bowel syndrome. *Gastroenterology* (submitted for publication).

Rao, S.S.C., Holdsworth, C.D. & Read, N.W. (1987) Anorectal sensitivity and reactivity in patients with ulcerative colitis. *Gastroenterology* **93**, 1270–1275.

Rao, S.S.C., Holdsworth, C.D. & Read, N.W. (1988a) Symptom and stool patterns in ulcerative colitis. *Gut* **29**, 342–345.

Rao, S.S.C., Read, N.W., Stobbard, J.H.H., Haines, W.G., Benjamin, S. & Holdsworth, C.D. (1988b) Anorectal contractility under basal conditions and during rectal infusion of saline in ulcerative colitis. *Gut* **29**, 769–777.

Read, N.W. (1986) Diarrhee motrice. In *Clinicals and Gastroenterology*, Vol. 15, pp. 657–686. W.B. Saunders, Philadelphia.

Richter, J.E., Barrage, C.F. & Castell, D.O. (1986) Abnormal sensory perception in patients with oesophageal chest pain. *Gastroenterology* **91**, 845–852.

Ritchie, J. (1973) Pain from distension of the pelvic colon by inflating a balloon in the irritable bowel syndrome. *Gut* **14**, 125–132.

Rumessen, J.J. & Goodman-Hayer, J. (1988) Functional bowel disease, malabsorption and abdominal distress after ingestion of fructose, sorbitol and fructose-sorbitol mixture. *Gastroenterology* **95**, 694–700.

Snape, W.J., Schiff, S. & Cohen, S. (1980) Effect of deoxycholic acid on colonic motility in the rabbit. *Am J Physiol* **288**, G321–G325.

Stanghellini, V., Camileri, M. & Malagelada, J-R. (1987) Chronic idiopathic intestinal pseudo-obstruction. Clinical and intestinal marometric findings. *Gut* 28, 5–12.

Sun, W.M., Read, N.W., Bannister, J.J., Shorthouse, A.T. & Donnelly, C.T. (1989) A common pathophysiology for full thickness rectal prolapse, anterior mucosal prolapse and solitary rectal ulcer. *Br J Surg* 76, 290–295.

Sun, W.M., Read, N.W. Prior, A., Daly, J., Cheah, S.K. & Grundy, D. (1990a) The sensory and motor responses to rectal distension vary according to rate and pattern of balloon inflation. *Gastroenterology* 99, 1008–1013.

Sun, W.M., Edwards, C.A., Rao, S.S.C., Prior, A. & Read, N.W. (1990b) The effect of nicardipine on anorectal motility in normal human volunteers and in patients with IBS. *Dig Dis Sci* 35, 885–890.

Swarbrick, E.T., Haggerty, J.E. & Bat, L. (1980) Site of pain from the irritable bowel syndrome. *Lancet* ii, 443–446.

Taylor, I., Darby, C., Hammond, P. & Highland, J. (1980) Effect of bile acid perfusion on colonic motor function in patients with the irritable bowel syndrome. *Scand J Gastroenterol* 15, 237–240.

Thaysen, E.H. & Pedersen, L. (1976) Idiopathic bile acid catharsis. *Gut* 17, 965–970.

Thompson, W.G., Dotterval, G., Drossman, D.A., Heaton, K.W. & Kruis, S.W. (1989) Irritable bowel syndrome: guidelines for the diagnosis. *Gastroenterol Int* 2, 92–95.

Welgan, P., Meshinpour, H. & Belar, M. (1988) The effect of anger on colon, motor and myoelectrical activity in the irritable bowel syndrome. *Gastroenterology* 94, 1150–1156.

White, A., Upton, A. & Collins, S.M. (1988) Is irritable bowel syndrome the asthma of the gut? *Gastroenterology* 94, A494.

Whitehead, W.E., Engel, B.T. & Schuster, M.M. (1980) Irritable bowel syndrome. Physiological and psychological differences between diarrhoea-predominant and constipation-predominant patients. *Dig Dis Sci* 25, 404–413.

Whitehead, W.E., Bosmatian, L., Zonderman, A.D. *et al.* (1988) Symptoms of psychologic distress associated with the irritable bowel syndrome. Comparison of community and medical clinical samples. *Gastroenterology* 95, 209–214.

Whorwell, P.J., Luppon, E.W., Erduran, D. & Wilson, K. (1986) Bladder smooth muscle dysfunction in patients with irritable bowel syndrome. *Gut* 27, 1014–1017.

Young, S.J., Alpers, D.H., Norland, C.C. *et al.* (1976) Psychiatric illness and the irritable bowel syndrome. Practical implications for the primary physician. *Gastroenterology* 70, 162–166.

Section 2
Motor Disturbance

2 *Disturbances in Colonic Motility*

N.W. Read

BASAL MOTOR ACTIVITY

Early studies suggested that colonic motor activity varied according to the predominant symptoms. Constipation was associated with an increase in segmental contractile activity, whereas diarrhoea was associated with a decrease in contractile activity. Thus, colonic motility was described as paradoxical (Almy, 1951; Connell, 1962; Wangel & Deller, 1965; Waller *et al.*, 1972); an excess of segmental contractions impaired the passage of colonic contents, while a reduction in this type of activity allowed the bowel contents to run free. More recent studies have shown the concept of paradoxical motility to be an oversimplification. First, colonic motor activity may be propulsive as well as segmenting in nature and, while an increase in segmenting activity would impair flow, if the motor activity was propulsive it would accelerate flow. Second, contractile activity can vary quite markedly from one site to the next. Recordings from the rectosigmoid region frequently show increased segmenting activity, whereas the motor activity a few centimetres on either side may be quite silent (Chowdhury *et al.*, 1976; Sun *et al.*, 1990). These observations suggest the existence of a rectosigmoid sphincter, which may control the delivery of the colonic contents into the rectum. Most early studies recorded from either a single sensor or a pair of sensors situated in the rectosigmoid regions and, as such, are not representative of the motor activity of the whole colon (Trotman & Misiewicz, 1988). Furthermore, the sensors may not have adequately distinguished between propagative and non-propagative contractions.

Multichannel myoelectrical and manometric recordings from the distal colon (Bueno *et al.*, 1980a, 1980b; Frexinos *et al.*, 1987), as far up as the splenic flexure, have shown that in patients who present with abdominal pain and constipation there is a preponderance of non-propulsive, short-spike bursts (Bueno *et al.*, 1980a, 1980b), which are probably the electrical counterpart of haustral contractions, and a reduction in migrating long-spike bursts, which are thought to be the electrical counterpart of the contractions that propel material through the colon. In contrast, those patients who present with diarrhoea, particularly painless diarrhoea, have a marked reduction in short-spike bursts but an increase in the frequency of the migrating long-spike bursts (Bueno *et al.*, 1980a; Frexinos *et al.*, 1987).

IS THERE A SPECIFIC MOTOR ABNORMALITY IN PATIENTS WITH IRRITABLE BOWEL SYNDROME?

About 15 years ago, at least two research groups (Snape *et al.*, 1976; Taylor *et al.*, 1978) reported an increased preponderance of three-cycle-a-minute myoelectrical activity in the rectosigmoid region in patients with IBS. This phenomenon was predominantly found in the constipated patients and could be associated with three-cycle-a-minute segmenting contractions (Snape *et al.*, 1977). However, not all research groups could demonstrate this abnormal finding. Latimer and his colleagues (Latimer *et al.*, 1981), in particular, showed that three-cycle-a-minute activity was no more common in patients with IBS than it was in psychoneurotic control subjects, or in otherwise normal control subjects. It is unlikely that Snape and Taylor were mistaken in their observations. What seems more probable is that there were crucial differences in the experimental design. These may include differences in the selection of patients, differences in the analysis of the recordings and differences in experimental technique. Upon reviewing all of the results from different centres in a recent symposium (Taylor, 1984), it appeared that those groups who had not used a bowel preparation recorded an abnormal preponderance of three-cycle-a-minute activity, whereas those who did use a bowel preparation failed to record this phenomenon. So does three-cycle-a-minute activity represent the response to distension with faecal material in a 'sensitized' and anxious patient?

Exaggerated responses to stimuli

Rectal distension

Several groups have shown that the rectum is abnormally reactive to distension. Relatively smaller volumes of air in a balloon give rise to repetitive phasic rectal contractions and more pronounced and precipitate internal sphincter relaxations (Whitehead *et al.*, 1980; Prior *et al.*, 1990, 1991). Rectal compliance is also markedly reduced. Enhanced reactivity to rectal distension is, however, only found in a subset of patients with IBS and is associated with increased rectal sensitivity (see Chapter 1).

Responses to meal ingestion

Ingestion of a meal normally induces an increase in colonic motility. Recent studies have demonstrated that this response is biphasic; an immediate response that is thought to be mediated by a neural reflex (Sun *et al.*, 1982; Glick *et al.*, 1984), but may be modulated by the release of cholecystokinin (Renny *et al.*, 1983); and a delayed response, that we have recently found to be associated with a rise in breath hydrogen (unpublished data), indicating the arrival of the first part of the meal in the colon. This so-called gastrocolonic response is more pronounced in patients with IBS (Kock *et al.*, 1968; Sun *et al.*, 1990) and is often associated with pain (Connell, 1962). Snape has also reported a delay in the gastrocolonic response in patients with IBS (Sullivan *et al.*, 1978). The mechanism for this delay is unclear. One possible explanation is that the delivery of the fatty test meal to a duodenal receptor site is delayed, although it is notable that gastric emptying of less nutrient-dense meals is not always delayed in IBS patients (Cann *et al.*, 1983; Narducci *et al.*, 1986).

Increased responsiveness to transmitter substances

Infusion of cholecystokinin results in an increase in colonic motor activity in patients with IBS compared with normal subjects and can reproduce symptoms of abdominal pain (Harvey & Read, 1973). Similarly, the cholinesterase inhibitor, neostigmine, causes an enhanced motor activity in patients with IBS compared with normal subjects and exacerbates abdominal pain (Chaudhary & Truelove, 1962).

Increased rectosigmoid response to stress

Thomas Almy observed changes in rectosigmoid motor activity in patients with IBS during emotionally charged interviews (Almy & Tulin, 1947). The motor response, however, appeared to be related to both the emotional response of the patient as well as to the predominant bowel habit. An angry response was associated with a marked increase in rectosigmoid activity and was much more likely to be found in patients with constipation and pain (Almy *et al.*, 1949, 1951). A tearful response was often associated with a reduction in colonic motor activity and was often found in patients who compained of diarrhoea (Welgan *et al.*, 1985).

CONCLUSIONS

Most studies suggest that although colonic motor disturbances are common in IBS, they are an exaggeration of the patterns seen in normal subjects rather than a specific abnormality. The case for a specific marker now seems dubious. The motor patterns may reflect the predominant bowel habit, more propulsive and less segmenting contractions being seen in patients with diarrhoea, the converse occurring in constipation. Particularly notable are the exaggerated responses to a variety of stimuli, food, distension, stress, chemicals. This hyperactivity could represent an increase in change in the properties of the smooth muscle, as well as an increase in bowel sensitivity (see Chapter 1).

REFERENCES

Almy, T.P. (1951) Experimental studies in the irritable bowel syndrome. *Am J Med* 10, 60–67.

Almy, T.P. & Tulin, M. (1947) Alterations in colonic function in man in health and distress: experimental production of changes stimulating the irritable bowel. *Gastroenterology* 8, 616–626.

Almy, T.P., Abbott, F.K. & Burrel, B. (1949) Alterations in colonic function in man in health and distress. III. Experimental production of sigmoid spasm in patients with spastic constipation. *Gastroenterology* 12, 437–449.

Almy, T.P., Abbott, F.K. & Hinkle, L.E. (1951) Alterations in colonic function in man in health and distress. IV. Hypomotility of the sigmoid colon and its relationship to the mechanism of functional diarrhoea. *Gastroenterology* 15, 95–103.

Bueno, L., Fioramonti, J., Frexinos, J. *et al.* (1980a) Colonic myoelectrical activity in diarrhoea and constipation. *Gastroenterology* 27, 381–389.

Bueno, L., Fioramonti, J., Ruckebusch, Y., Frexinos, J. & Coulom, P. (1980b) Evaluation of colonic myoelectric activity in health and functional disorders. *Gut* 21, 480–485.

Cann, P.A., Read, N.W., Brown, C., Hobson, N. & Holdsworth, C.D. (1983) The irritable bowel syndrome (IBS): relationship of disorders in the transit of a single solid meal to symptom patterns. *Gut* 24, 405–411.

Chaudhary, N.A. & Truelove, S.C. (1962) Human colonic motility: comparative study of normal subjects, patients with ulcerative colitis and patients with the irritable bowel syndrome. II. The effect of prostigmine. *Gastroenterology* 40, 18–26.

Chowdhury, A.R., Dinoso, D.P. & Lorber, S.H. (1976) Characterization of a hyperactive segment of the rectosigmoid junction. *Gastroenterology* 71, 584–588.

Connell, A.M. (1962) The motility of the pelvic colon II. Paradoxical motility in diarrhoea and constipation. *Gut* 3, 342–348.

Frexinos, J., Fioramonti, J. & Bueno, L. (1987) Colonic myoelectrical activity in IBS painless diarrhoea. *Gut* 28, 1613–1618.

Glick, M.E., Meshkinpour, H., Holderman, S. *et al.* (1984) Colonic dysfunction in patients with thoracic spinal cord injury. *Gastroenterology* 86, 287–294.

Harvey, R.F. & Read, A.E. (1973) Effect of cholecystokinin on colonic motility in symptoms in patients with the irritable bowel syndrome. *Lancet* i, 1–3.

Kock, N.G., Hulten, L. & Leandoer, L. (1968) A study of motility in different parts of the human colon. Resting activity, response to feeding and to prostigmine. *Scand J Gastroenterol* 3, 163–169.

Latimer, P., Sarna, S., Campbell, D. *et al.* (1981) Colonic motor and myoelectrical activity: a comparison study of subjects, psychoneurotic patients and patients with the irritable bowel syndrome. *Gastroenterology* 80, 893–901.

Narducci, F., Bassotti, G. & Renarta, N.T. (1986) Colonic motility in gastric emptying in patients with irritable bowel syndrome. *Dig Dis Sci* 31, 241–246.

Prior, A., Maxton, D.G. & Whorwell, P.J. (1990) Anorectal manometry in irritable bowel syndrome: differences between diarrhoea- and constipation-predominant subjects. *Gut* (in press)

Prior, A., Sorial, E., Sun, W.M. & Read, N.W. (1991) Rectal sensitivity: a rational means of categorizing patients with the irritable bowel syndrome. (submitted to Gastroenterology).

Renny, A., Snape, W.J. & Sun, E.A. (1983) Role of cholecystokinin in the gastro-colonic response to a meal. *Gastroenterology* **85**, 17–21.

Snape, W.J., Carlsson, G.M., Cohen, S. (1976) Colonic myoelectrical activity in the irritable bowel syndrome. *Gastroenterology* **70**, 326–330.

Snape, W.J., Carlsson, G.M., Motarazzo, S.A. *et al.* (1977) Evidence that abnormal myoelectrical activity produces colonic motor dysfunction in the irritable bowel syndrome. *Gastroenterology* **72**, 383–387.

Sullivan, M.A., Cohen, S. & Snape, W.J. (1978) Colonic myoelectrical activity in the irritable bowel syndrome. *New Engl J Med* **298**, 878–883.

Sun, E.A., Snape, W.J. & Cohen, S. (1982) The role of opiate receptors and cholinergic neurones in the gastrocolonic response. *Gastroenterology* **82**, 689–693.

Sun, W.M., Edwards, C.A., Prior, A., Rao, S.S.C. & Read, N.W. (1990) The effect of nicardipine on anorectal motility in normal human volunteers and patients with IBS. *Dig Dis Sci* **35**, 885–890.

Taylor, I. (1984) Colonic motility in the irritable bowel syndrome. In Read N.W. (ed), *Irritable Bowel Syndrome*, pp. 89–104. Grune & Stratton, London.

Taylor, I., Derby, C. & Hammond, P. (1978) Is there a myoelectrical abnormality in the irritable bowel syndrome? *Gut* **19**, 391–395.

Trotman, I.F. & Misiewicz, J.J. (1988) Sigmoid motility in diverticular disease and the irritable bowel syndrome. *Gut* **22**, 218–222.

Waller, S.L., Misiewicz, J.J. & Kiley, N. (1972) Effect of eating on motility of the pelvic colon in constipation and diarrhoea. *Gut* **13**, 805–811.

Wangel, A.G. & Deller, D.J. (1965) Intestinal motility in man. III. Mechanisms of constipation and diarrhoea with particular reference to the irritable colon syndrome. *Gastroenterology* **48**, 69–84.

Welgan, P., Meshinpour, H. & Hoehler, F. (1985) The effect of stress on colonic and electrical activity in irritable bowel syndrome. *Psychosom Med* **47**, 139–149.

Whitehead, W.E., Engel, B.T. & Schuster, M.M. (1980) Irritable bowel syndrome; physiological and psychological differences between diarrhoea-predominant and constipation-predominant patients. *Dig Dis Sci* **25**, 404–413.

3 Small Bowel Motor Activity: A Key to Understanding Functional Disorders of the Bowel

D.L. Wingate

The term 'functional bowel disorder' is often used as a shorthand by physicians for a patient who is mad or hypochondriac, but functional does not mean imaginary or non-existent. Functional disorder simply means disordered function. A functional disorder is due to pathophysiology which is a consequence of unidentified pathology. As soon as we can identify the pathology, it is removed from the list of functional disorders. For example, should we find that all non-ulcer dyspepsia is due to *Helicobacter*, we would call this *Helicobacter* gastritis; the terms non-ulcer dyspepsia or functional dyspepsia would disappear, so the word 'functional' means in effect that we recognize that there is a problem but we cannot explain it.

INNERVATION OF THE GUT

Until recently, the gut was thought to be innervated by parasympathetic nerves, which stimulate motility, and sympathetic nerves, which inhibit it. This is incorrect. Gastrointestinal smooth muscle is innervated by enteric neurones arising from the plexuses within the gut wall and these plexuses are collectively known as the enteric nervous system (ENS). The extrinsic parasympathetic or sympathetic nerves modulate this local command system. The ENS contains the myenteric or Auerbach's plexus between the longitudinal and circular muscle layers, and plexus of Meissner between the circular muscle and the mucosa; these two plexuses invest the entire bowel from the oesophagus to the anus. One of the striking things about the ENS is its peculiar resemblance to the cerebral cortex. The ENS has as many neurones as the spinal cord; it consists of ganglia connected by a network of interconnecting directional axons; it contains a profusion of potential neurotransmitters and neuromodulators; there is a blood–ENS barrier, like the blood–brain barrier; and above all there is a functional resemblance between the organization of gut function by the ENS, and the control of movement by the central nervous system (CNS).

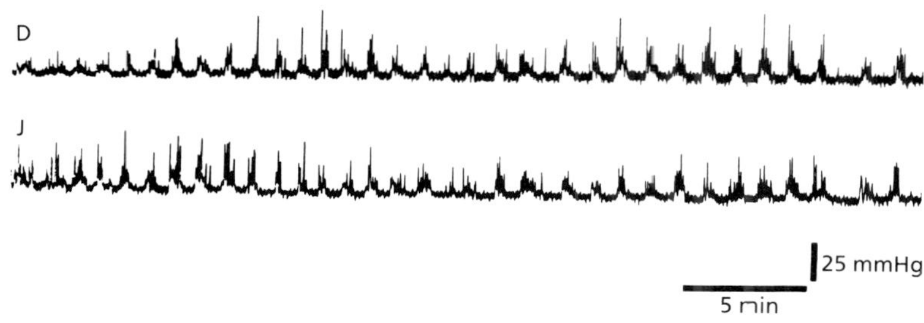

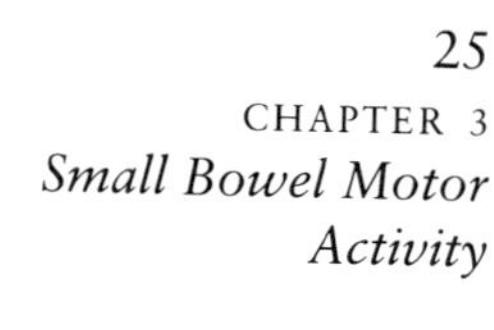

Fig. 3.1. Clustered contractions during phase II fasting activity recorded in both duodenum (D) and jejunum (J) in a patient with IBS.

It is easier to investigate the function of the ENS by studying motor activity: the sensory side of the ENS is extremely difficult to study, and methods for studying absorption or secretion do not possess adequate temporal resolution.

MIGRATING MOTOR COMPLEX

The migrating motor complex (MMC) is a well described and characterized pattern of motor activity, which is orchestrated by the ENS. It consists of three phases: a period of quiescence (phase I), a period of contractile activity which is irregular in amplitude and frequency (phase II), and a brief phase of regular contractions (phase III). Phase III activity is a remarkably constant activity. It is seen in virtually all the mammalian species, although in carnivores which eat discrete meals it occurs only during fasting. In our 24-hour studies of normal people, fasting motor activity occurs for about 16 hours out of 24. In ruminants, it occurs all the time and food appears to be conveyed along the small intestine in batches separated by sequential phase IIIs. The MMC appears to be a motor pattern which is programmed entirely by the ENS. Moreover, contrary to published data, we have found no relationship between the MMC and the sleep cycle. We do not think that the ENS is simply cycling with the CNS; the evidence is that the resting activities of the brain and gut are independent. When we eat a meal, the MMC is immediately switched off and replaced by irregular postprandial activity. The switching of patterns takes place at a similar time at all levels of the bowel, so it is probably not purely dependent on local luminal contact with food.

Recently we have found that the rectum also appears to have a similar biorhythm which is only really marked during sleep (Kumar *et al.*, 1990); bursts of 8–10 powerful contractions occur at a steady rhythm of three per minute and are separated by periods of 50–60 minutes. Recent data shows that the rectal motor complex is not temporally related to the small intestinal MMC.

LINKAGE WITH THE ENTERIC AND CENTRAL NERVOUS SYSTEMS

The phrase 'gut brain' is useful because it seems a reasonable description of a nerve network that can take in sensory information from sensory receptors, integrate this information, and select programmes of activity. The 'gut brain' is not, however, completely autonomous. There is an important link between the brain and the ENS, with most of the traffic running from the gut to the brain. About 90% of the fibres in the vagus are afferent. Much of the amount of information that goes up to the brain is not perceived, but may trigger subconscious responses in the gut or other parts of the body. The 5000 or so efferent vagal fibres synapse with about 50 million enteric neurones, suggesting modulatory rather than direct control of gastrointestinal function.

There are several examples of how the brain may modulate gut motor activity. During sleep, the MMC cycles more frequently, its rate of propagation is slower and a phase II activity is absent or very much reduced (Kellow *et al.*, 1990). Experimental stress can perturb the MMC patterns by prolonging the duration between phase IIIs (McRae *et al.*, 1982).

MOTOR PATTERNS IN IRRITABLE BOWEL SYNDROME PATIENTS

The most common small bowel abnormality in irritable bowel syndrome (IBS) patients consists of prolonged periods of clusters of

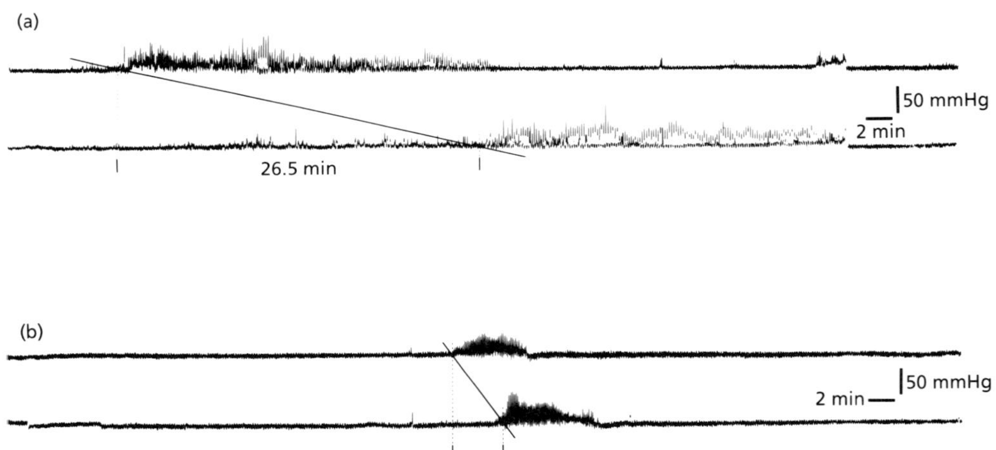

Fig. 3.2. (a) Manometric recording of a jejunal MMC in the IBS patient. (b) For comparison, a jejunal MMC in a normal subject. Both recordings were made during sleep. In each case the sensors were 15 cm apart from the orad sensor located just distal to the duodenojejunal flexure. Note the prolongation of phase III and its slow migration in the patient.

contractions occuring at a frequency of about one a minute in the small bowel (Fig. 3.1) (Kellow & Phillips, 1987; Kellow *et al.*, 1990) Clusters of contractions also occur in normal people but rarely for longer than 10 minutes. These clustered contractions are seen in freely ambulant subjects (Kellow *et al.*, 1990) but are also evoked by stress (Kumar & Wingate, 1985).

Clusters of contractions occur during the day; they are uncommon at night when patients are asleep. Such patients may have a neurotic bowel (an abnormal preponderance of a normal pattern), probably due to increased influence of the CNS on ENS activity; when the CNS activity is reduced during sleep, the abnormal pattern disappears or is much reduced.

An abnormal pattern that occurs at night is highly suggestive of an enteric nervous disorder. Figure 3.2 shows a phase III which is nearly 30 minutes long, moving at one-fifth of the speed of a normal phase III. This pattern is almost certainly indicative of an enteric neuropathy.

A CLASSIFICATION OF FUNCTIONAL SMALL INTESTINAL MOTOR DISORDERS

One method of classifying the motor disorders that we see in IBS is to divide them into CNS-dependent and CNS-independent disorders. Chronic idiopathic intestinal pseudo-obstruction is CNS-independent. Most cases show abnormal MMC configuration and migration (Stanghellini *et al.*, 1987) and the abnormal motor patterns persist during sleep.

Abnormal motor activity that is present only when the subject is awake is termed CNS-dependent; the ENS may not be damaged but simply subjected to a bombardment of information from the CNS, as might occur, for example, during stress. The function of the ENS may be appropriate, but the demands made on it may be inappropriate.

Another form of CNS-dependent motor disturbance exists where there is normal CNS activity but the ENS has been damaged or sensitized by exposure to bacterial products. The problem is still the CNS dependence, as far as we know, because these people only exhibit disorders during the day; the simple process of waking up and having to do things is enough to knock an unstable ENS off balance.

REFERENCES

Kellow, J.E. & Phillips, S.F. (1987) Altered small bowel motility in irritable bowel syndrome is correlated with symptoms. *Gastroenterology* 92, 1885–1893.

Kellow, J.E., Gill, R.C. & Wingate, D.L. (1990) Prolonged ambulant recordings of small bowel motility demonstrate abnormalities in the irritable bowel syndrome. *Gastroenterology* 98, 1208–1218.

Kumar, D. & Wingate, D.L. (1985) The irritable bowel syndrome; a paroxysmal motor disorder. *Lancet* **2**, 973–977.

Kumar, D., Thompson, P.D. & Wingate, D.L. (1990) Absence of synchrony between the human rectal motor complex (RMC), and the migrating motor complex (MMC). *Am J Physiol* **258**. G

McRae, S., Younger, K., Thompson., D.G. & Wingate, D.L. (1982) Sustained mental stress alters human jejunal motor activity. *Gut* **23**, 404–409.

Stanghellini, V., Camilleri, M. & Malagelada, J-R. (1987) Chronic intestinal pseudo-obstruction: clinical and manometric findings. *Gut* **28**, 5–12.

4 *Abnormalities of Gastroduodenal Motility*

V. Stanghellini

INTRODUCTION

Irritable bowel syndrome (IBS) is the commonest gastrointestinal syndrome in Western countries (Almy, 1983). It represents a part of the large añ loosely defined group of disorders characterized by symptoms attributable to derangements of digestive functions in the absence of organic and systemic diseases. This group also includes idiopathic dyspepsia (ID) and chronic idiopathic intestinal pseudo-obstruction (CIIP). The nosologic borderlines in this area are difficult to draw. Some believe all the conditions represent the expression of a common pathogenetic mechanism acting at different levels of the digestive canal with variable degrees of severity (Read, 1987). The type of symptoms seen in functional digestive syndromes, and particularly epigastric fullness, vomiting, abdominal bloating, constipation and diarrhoea, suggest that they may be due to abnormal gastrointestinal motility.

Important technical improvements have allowed, in recent years, a broader knowledge of the motor activities in all regions of the digestive canal. This has led to the recognition of gastrointestinal motor abnormalities in a number of pathological conditions, including functional syndromes. However, no specific pathophysiologic markers have been identified in any of these functional syndromes and, consequently, they are still classified only by their symptoms, and their diagnosis remains one of exclusion.

DEFINITION AND DIAGNOSIS OF FUNCTIONAL GASTROINTESTINAL SYNDROMES

A standardized diagnostic nomenclature of functional gastrointestinal disorders is needed both for research purposes and for clinical practice. Many confusing definitions have been published over the years, but gastroenterologists are currently making an effort to achieve a more rational framework.

Intestinal pseudo-obstruction

Intestinal pseudo-obstruction was first firmly defined by Maldonado and colleagues (Maldonado *et al.*, 1970) as a syndrome characterized by symptoms and signs resembling those of mechanical obstruction in the absence of a mechanical obstacle to intestinal transit. It may be acute (AIP: when the obstructive episode is self-limiting) or chronic (CIP: when episodes tend to relapse). It is caused by impaired transit of intestinal contents due to inappropriate motility. Two main types of CIP are recognized: myogenic and neurogenic. In the former, smooth muscle cells are affected and transit is impaired because of reduced strength of contractility; in the latter, abnormalities of extrinsic and/or intrinsic nervous control systems cause severe uncoordination of digestive contractions (Stanghellini *et al.*, 1988a). Both myogenic and neurogenic CIP can be secondary to a number of organic or systemic diseases (Stanghellini *et al.*, 1988a) or idiopathic, when no possible cause is recognized. During pseudo-obstructive episodes, CIP can be easily confused with mechanical obstruction, while, between episodes, patients generally complain of a variety of digestive symptoms which resemble severe dyspepsia or IBS. In both instances differential diagnoses must be based upon the clinical history as well as radiologic, endoscopic and biochemical findings (Stanghellini *et al.*, 1988a). Measurements of gastrointestinal motility may be helpful in differentiating functional from mechanical obstruction (Malagelada & Stanghellini, 1985; Stanghellini *et al.*, 1988a), but, as will be discussed in greater detail below, it does not clearly separate CIP from severe dyspepsia and IBS.

Irritable bowel syndrome

Irritable bowel syndrome still defies a strict definition (Malagelada & Camilleri, 1985), but a general agreement exists in indicating that it is a syndrome characterized by periodic or chronic symptoms of diarrhoea, constipation and abdominal pain (Harrison, 1987). Questionnaires have been used to obtain 'objective' quantifications of symptoms in IBS patients and to differentiate the functional syndrome from abdominal pain and/or changes in bowel movements due to organic diseases (Manning *et al.*, 1978; Kruis *et al.*, 1984). Symptoms such as alternating bowel habit (constipation/diarrhoea), particularly when associated with abdominal pain and flatulence, lasting longer than 2 years, are strongly indicative of the functional syndrome. Abdominal distension, change of pain with bowel movements, mucus in the stools and a sensation of incomplete evacuation are common in IBS patients, but are also common in other conditions involving the colon, such as ulcerative colitis. The combination of detailed history taking and simple laboratory tests allows the correct diagnosis to be established in the vast majority of patients (Kruis *et al.*, 1984).

Dyspepsia

Many definitions of dyspepsia have been proposed over the last few decades. Some of them tend to hybridize the concept of dyspepsia with that of IBS. In 1968, for example, Rhind and Watson coined the term 'flatulent dyspepsia' to indicate a syndrome characterized by 'epigastric discomfort after meals, a feeling of fullness so that tight clothing is loosened, eructation, with temporary relief and regurgitation of sour liquid into the mouth, and heartburn' (Rhind & Watson, 1968). More recently, efforts have been made to differentiate ID from IBS (Colin-Jones *et al.*, 1988; Barbara *et al.*, 1989). We defined dyspepsia as 'episodic or persistent abdominal symptoms, often related to feeding, which patients or physicians believe to be due to disorders of the proximal portions of the digestive canal; consequently, ID is defined as dyspepsia which is not attributable to structural, drug-induced, alcohol-induced or metabolic disease, but is thought to be related to disorders of upper gut function or to abnormalities of a patient's perception of normal function' (Barbara *et al.*, 1989). The main symptoms occurring in patients with ID are upper abdominal pain and/or discomfort, postprandial fullness, early satiety or inability to finish a normal meal, anorexia, belching, nausea and heartburn. Associated symptoms such as postprandial drowsiness and headache are also common in ID patients. The diagnosis of ID, like IBS, is based on attentive history taking and exclusion of possible organic or systemic causes of the symptoms by appropriate investigation (Barbara *et al.*, 1989). No physiopathological markers of ID or IBS have been identified so far.

GASTROINTESTINAL MOTILITY IN FUNCTIONAL DIGESTIVE DISORDERS

As previously mentioned, symptoms of functional digestive syndromes are suggestive of derangements of gastrointestinal motor activities. Specifically, symptoms characteristic of IBS and colonic pseudo-obstruction are suggestive of motor abnormalities of the distal portions of the bowel (changes in bowel habits, diffuse abdominal pain and bloating), while ID and proximal CIP are characterized by symptoms suggesting motor abnormalities of the stomach and adjacent portions of the gut (epigastric pain, postprandial fullness, early satiety, anorexia, nausea, vomiting, belching, heartburn and regurgitation). For this reason, most of the studies carried out so far have investigated electromechanical motor events in the colon and rectum of IBS patients (Connel, 1962; Snape *et al.*, 1976, 1977; Taylor *et al.*, 1978; Bueno *et al.*, 1980) and in the stomach and small bowel in patients with ID (Telander, 1978; Rees *et al.*, 1980; You *et al.*, 1980, 1981; Malagelada & Stanghellini, 1985; Camilleri *et al.*, 1986a; Labò *et al.*, 1986). Only a handful of studies have evaluated digestive motor functions in CIP due to the limited number of patients affected by this severe syndrome (Stanghellini *et al.*, 1988a).

We will very briefly summarize the present knowledge of gastroduodenal motor patterns in ID and CIP and we will also present the scanty data existing in IBS patients, together with some experiences obtained in our laboratory.

Gastrointestinal motility in idiopathic dyspepsia

Isolated reports of postprandial antral hypomotility (Rees *et al.*, 1980) and disruption of basal electrical rhythm of antral smooth muscle cells (Telander *et al.*, 1978; You *et al.*, 1980, 1981) have been the subject of reports since the beginning of the 1980s. More recently, a systematic study was carried out to measure fasting and postprandial gastrointestinal motility in 104 patients affected by unexplained digestive symptoms seen consecutively at the Mayo Clinic (Malagelada & Stanghellini, 1985). Inclusion criteria were not excessively strict. Two of the following symptoms were required for entry to the study; unexplained nausea, vomiting and upper abdominal pain for at least 3 months. Patients also complained of numerous other symptoms, some of which were not directly referrable to the proximal portions of the gut, such as diarrhoea ($\approx 20\%$) and constipation ($\approx 15\%$). A clear-cut distinction between IBS and ID was not attempted. Gastrointestinal manometry failed to detect any abnormality in 21 individuals; eight subjects had normal motility disturbed by sharp increases in intra-abdominal pressure which caused rumination; 72 exhibited antral hypomotility, either isolated ($\approx 40\%$), or in combination with disordered intestinal mobility ($\approx 30\%$). In the group of 32 patients with both gastric and intestinal dysmobility, three different intestinal motor abnormalities were identified.

1 Bursts of non-propagated phasic pressure activity during fasting were observed in 13 patients (41%). Bursts were defined as periods lasting at least 2 minutes of continuous high amplitude (>20 mmHg) and high frequency (10–12/minute) phasic contractions, which were non-propagated and not followed by motor quiescence (unlike typical phase III of the interdigestive migrating motor complex (IDMMC). Phasic contractions were often superimposed upon tonic elevations of the baseline.

2 Abnormal activity fronts (phase III) of the IDMMC, which were associated with bursts, were observed in 13 patients (41%). Both propagation and configuration of activity fronts could be abnormal. Aberrant propagation was defined as the simultaneous or retro-

grade appearance of an activity front over at least a 30 cm segment of small bowel. Aberrant configuration was defined as intense (>30 mmHg) and prolonged (>3 minutes duration) tonic elevations of baseline pressure during propagation of the activity front through one or more levels of the small bowel.

3 Inability of meal ingestion to convert fasting into fed motor patterns was observed in six patients (18%). In all cases fasting motor patterns were clearly abnormal and were not modified after food ingestion.

No correlation was found between the type of symptoms reported by patients and the type of motor abnormalities recorded, nor between the symptoms and the presence of motor abnormalities. This was not altogether unexpected since severe gastroparesis may be encountered sporadically in asymptomatic patients with insulin-dependent diabetes (Feldman *et al.*, 1984). Moreover, approximately 50% of patients with unexplained dyspeptic symptoms have normal gastric emptying times (Stanghellini *et al.*, 1988b). Despite the fact that an association indeed exists between ID and gastrointestinal motor abnormalities in some patients, the pathogenesis of dyspeptic symptoms remains unknown. It has been suggested that stress may play a role in susceptible individuals. Stressful stimuli applied to healthy individuals have been shown to induce postprandial antral hypomotility and possibly also disruption of fed motor patterns, with the appearance of activity front-like activities in the proximal small bowel (Thompson *et al.*, 1982; Stanghellini *et al.*, 1983). These motor abnormalities, which may be mediated by adrenergic and opioid transmitters (Stanghellini *et al.*, 1983, 1984; Camilleri *et al.*, 1986b), are strikingly similar to those spontaneously present in patients with dyspeptic symptoms. A considerable amount of anecdotal evidence supports the commonly held belief that stressful life-events play an important role in the development of gastro-intestinal symptoms (Lagarde & Spiro, 1984; Thompson, 1984). It would be tempting to speculate that the gastrointestinal motor ab-normalities seen in dyspeptic patients are induced by environmental stress. However, experimental provocation of motor abnormalities in healthy subjects by stressful stimuli rarely elicits any symptoms (Talley & Piper, 1986).

In the light of all these considerations, the relation between gastrointestinal motor abnormalities and dyspeptic symptoms cannot be reduced to a simple cause–effect phenomenon.

Gastrointestinal motility in chronic idiopathic intestinal pseudo-obstruction

The first systematic study was of intestinal motility in CIIP were carried out in 42 patients with CIIP, seen consecutively at the Mayo Clinic (Stanghellini *et al.*, 1987). Thirty-three of the 42 patients had previously undergone abdominal surgery: 12 laparatomy alone, 10 gastric surgery (including vagotomy), seven segmental small bowel resection, and four colectomy with ileoproctostomy. Gastric motility was found to be reduced in all the patients in whom antral recording was technically possible. All patients also showed clear evidence of intestinal dysmotility. Four abnormal motor patterns were recognized in the proximal small bowel: aberrant activity fronts, abnormal bursts, inability of meal ingestion to convert fasting into fed motor patterns, and sustained (for over 30 minutes) and intense phasic pressure activity at one recording site, with normal or reduced pressure activity at other levels of the intestine. No apparent relationship was found between the four abnormal manometric patterns observed and the previous surgical procedures, nor between these patterns and the type or severity of symptoms. Over 80% of the patients had at least two abnormal manometric features; almost one-third of the patients exhibited all the manometric abnormalities.

Gastrointestinal motility characterized by powerful but disorganized contractions is indicative of preserved myogenic activity, but abnormal neurogenic control. This has been confirmed both in animal models and in human studies. Mice with genetically transmitted depletion of enteric neurones show frequent powerful phasic contractions superimposed upon tonic spasms of the intestinal walls (Wood, 1973). Patients with orthostatic hypotension due to generalized autonomic failure were shown to present severe motor abnormalities very similar to those observed in neurogenic CIIP, such as abnormal activity fronts, bursts and sustained uncoordinated hypermotility (Camilleri *et al.*, 1985).

Manometric gastrointestinal recordings are very different in patients with preserved nervous control but with damaged smooth muscle. If the muscular damage is incomplete, motility will be represented by normally coordinated but weak contractions. No contractions can be recorded in patients with more severe impairments of muscular contractility (Stanghellini *et al.*, 1988a; Malagelada *et al.*, 1986). Motility records can also be useful to differentiate mechanical from 'functional' intestinal obstructions. Myoelectric studies in experimental animals (Summers *et al.*, 1983) as well as manometric recordings in patients (Malagelada *et al.*, 1986) have clearly demonstrated that intestinal mechanical obstruction triggers the onset of characteristic 'clusters' of contractions or myoelectrical spike bursts in the portions of the small bowel proximal to the occlusion, both during fasting and after feeding. Clusters are replaced by weak, irregular contractions in long-term mechanical obstruction, when smooth muscle cells lose their contractile force. Postprandial clusters are suggestive of mechanical obstruction. Discrete clustered contractions are also possible components of phase II of the IDMMC in healthy individuals and are particularly frequent in IBS patients (Kellow & Phillips, 1987). They may be mediated via cholinergic pathways since infusions of neostigmine, an anticholinesterase agent, have been reported to elicit jejunal clustered contractions more frequently in IBS patients than asymptomatic controls (Kellow *et al.*, 1988).

Gastrointestinal motility in irritable bowel syndrome

The causes of IBS have long been attributed to abnormal motility of the large bowel and many studies have been carried out to investigate this function in basal conditions and after different stimuli (Snape *et al.*, 1976; Sullivan *et al.*, 1978; Latimer *et al.*, 1981). More recently, some attention has been paid to the role that small bowel motility may play in this syndrome (Kumar & Wingate, 1985; Kellow & Phillips, 1987; Kellow *et al.*, 1988). Moreover, possible extraintestinal causes of IBS have been the subject of research in recent years (Whorwell *et al.*, 1981, 1986a; Smart *et al.*, 1986). Colonic, small intestinal and extraintestinal features of IBS are discussed in greater detail elsewhere in this book. Very little is known of gastric and duodenal motility in IBS.

The typical symptoms of IBS (Manning *et al.*, 1978; Kruis *et al.*, 1984) are not suggestive of deranged gastroduodenal motility. Nevertheless, patients with this syndrome quite often complain of characteristic dyspeptic symptoms such as nausea and vomiting, epigastric fullness and inability to finish a normal meal (Whorwell *et al.*, 1986b). No systematic study has been carried out to evaluate gastroduodenal motility in IBS patients with or without dyspeptic symptoms. Indirect measurements of gastrointestinal motility have been obtained by studying gastric emptying times by radioisotopic techniques, but results in IBS patients were often normal (Acharya *et al.*, 1983). In 1983, Acharya and colleagues stated, 'future studies on abnormalities in IBS should investigate other aspects of gastric motor functions', but no such studies have ever been published.

Between September 1985 and September 1988, we performed 225 gastroduodeno-jejunal manometries in our laboratory at the University of Bologna. Of these, 71 were obtained from patients with unexplained gastrointestinal syndromes: seven CIIP (four male, three female, 15–61 years); eight IBS (three male, five female, 15–65 years); 30 prominent ID (12 male, 18 female, 22–63 years); and 26 prominent IBS and ID (two male, 24 female, 19–71 years). Idiopathic dyspepsia and CIIP were defined as reported above and previously published (Barbara *et al.*, 1989; Stanghellini *et al.*, 1987). Diagnosis of IBS was based on criteria proposed by Manning *et al.* (1978) and Kruis *et al.* (1984). Specifically, two main symptoms were required: irregularity of bowel movements (constipation, diarrhoea, alternating bowel movements), and abdominal pain (possibly relieved by bowel movements). Associated symptoms were: abdominal distension, flatulence, sensation of incomplete evacuation. Most of the patients had both IBS and ID. The two syndromes were equally severe in 26 patients, IBS was prominent in eight, and ID in 30 patients.

We compared gastrointestinal motor patterns in IBS patients (with and without associated ID) with those in patients with prominent ID and in eight asymptomatic volunteers (four male, four female, 28–50 years), who served as healthy controls.

Gastroduodeno-jejunal motility was recorded by a low-compliance perfusion system attached to a multi-lumen, open-tipped tube with 5–6 recording sites positioned across the antroduodenal junction (1 cm apart) and 2–3 recording sites in the proximal small bowel (10–20 cm apart). Recordings were performed with patients off medication for at least 48 hours, after an overnight fast, and both under fasting conditions (180–500 minutes, median: 240 minutes) and after ingestion of a 613 kcal meal containing digestible solids (40–180 minutes; median 120 minutes). Tracings were analysed visually. Frequency and intensity of antral contractions were quantified both during fasting and after feeding. Motility indexes (MI = number of waves × sum of amplitudes) were computed at 10-minute intervals. The relative durations of the motor phases of the IDMMC were quantified. The number and type of abnormal motor patterns were also analysed. Idiopathic dyspepsia, IBS and IBS+ID patients presented several gastrointestinal motor abnormalities compared to healthy controls. Antral hypomotility was detected during fasting and after feeding in the majority of patients: 70% in ID patients, 63% in IBS patients and 49% (fasting) and 77% (after feeding) in IBS+ID patients (Fig. 4.1). The duration of interdigestive motor phases recorded in the proximal small bowel also appeared abnormal in all three groups of patients, as depicted in Fig. 4.2. Periods of fasting uncoordinated motility (phase II) were longer in ID (84% ± 13%; mean ± standard deviation), IBS (81% ± 9%) and IBS+ID patients (84% ± 12%) compared to asymptomatic controls (67% ± 21%). Periods of motor quiescence (phase I) were correspondingly shorter in ID (11% ± 12%), IBS (6% ± 6%) and IBS+ID patients (11% ± 11%), compared with controls (27% ± 19%). Relatively high percentages of patients presented abnormal motor patterns in the proximal small bowel. Abnormal activity fronts and abnormal bursts of activity were observed respectively in 17 and 20% of ID patients, 13 and 25% of IBS patients and 15 and 39% of IBS+ID patients. Sustained contractions and inability of meal ingestion to convert fast into fed motor pattern were not detected in any of the patients we examined. Two main considerations can be drawn from these results.

1 Motor abnormalities of the gastric antrum and of the proximal tracts of the small bowel can be found in a high proportion of

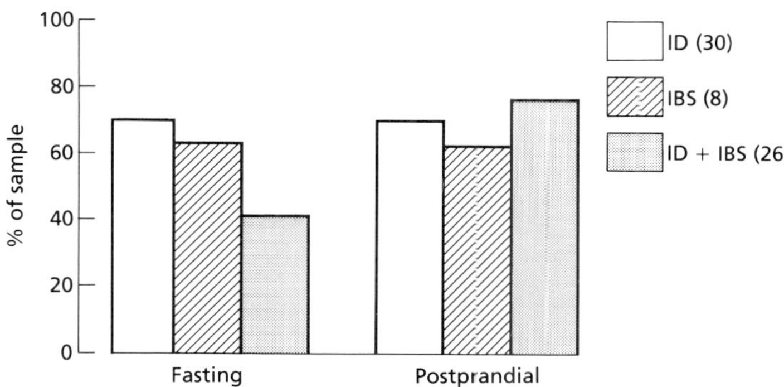

Fig. 4.1. Frequency of fasting and postprandial antral hypomotility in patients with idiopathic dyspepsia (ID) and irritable bowel syndrome (IBS) alone or in combination.

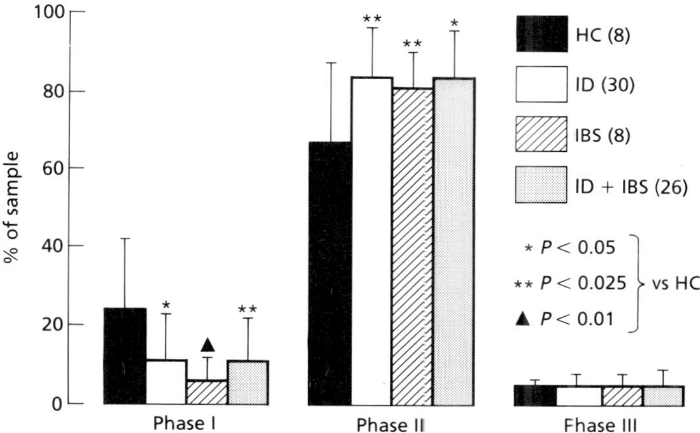

Fig. 4.2. Duration of intestinal interdigestive motor phases in patients with idiopathic dyspepsia (ID) and irritable bowel syndrome (IBS) alone or in combination. HC = healthy controls.

patients with IBS, regardless of the severity of associated dyspeptic symptoms.

2 There is no apparent relationship between the manometric patterns recorded and the type or severity of symptoms.

Figure 4.3 shows the frequency of intestinal abnormal motor patterns detected in the present study, compared to those of a group of CIIP patients previously investigated by an identical technique (Stanghellini *et al.*, 1987). As might have been expected, less severe disruption of the motor functions of proximal portions of the digestive canal were observed in patients with prominent IBS. The present results need to be confirmed in larger groups of patients, although they are not altogether unexpected since, as previously

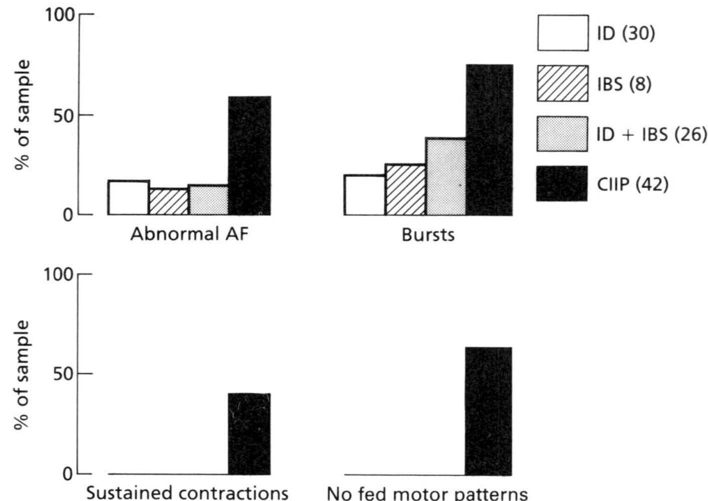

Fig. 4.3. Frequency of intestinal abnormal motor patterns in patients with idiopathic dyspepsia (ID), irritable bowel syndrome (IBS) and chronic idiopathic intestinal pseudo-obstruction (CIIP).

mentioned, functional digestive symptoms are not predictive of any particular motor abnormality so far noticed in the stomach and proximal small bowel (Malagelada & Stanghellini, 1985; Stanghellini *et al.*, 1987).

On the contrary, some motor abnormalities of more distal portions of the digestive canal seem to have a more direct relationship with IBS symptoms. Kumar and Wingate reported that 10 out of 30 episodes of abnormal jejunal motility recorded in 22 IBS patients were associated with abdominal discomfort (Sullivan *et al.*, 1978). Kellow and Phillips observed that over 60% of ileal prolonged propagated contractions were associated with cramping abdominal pain in IBS patients; however, only 17% of these powerful contractions of the distal bowel elicited symptoms in healthy subjects (Kellow & Phillips, 1987). The reasons for this discrepancy between patients and controls are not clear. Evidently, this particular motor pattern is not sufficient *per se* to elicit the onset of symptoms. A 'predisposed environment' appears to be necessary.

A further consideration on the relationship between symptoms and motor functions derives from the frequencies of abnormal patterns detected in the three groups of patients in this study, and of the CIP patients previously described (Stanghellini *et al.*, 1987). Idiopathic dyspepsia, IBS and IBS+ID patients presented approximately similar frequencies of aberrant activity fronts, ranging from 13% (IBS) to 17% (IBS+ID), while this motor abnormality was markedly more frequent in CIP patients (50%). Bursts were progressively more frequent in ID (20%), IBS (25%), IBS+ID (39%), and CIP (75%). Furthermore, sustained contractions and inability of the meal to convert fasting into fed motility were not detected in ID, IBS and IBS+ID, but were present respectively in 40 and 64% of CIP patients. A certain relationship between the severity of clinical manifestations and gastroduodenal motor abnormalities seems, therefore, to exist: the frequency of these motor abnormalities being higher in the most severe syndromes.

CONCLUSIONS

Definitions of functional digestive syndromes are still controversial and, in the absence of pathophysiologic markers, they are based merely upon symptoms (Maldonado *et al.*, 1970; Barbara *et al.*, 1986; Harrison, 1987).

Many uncertainties remain regarding the reasons why some patients mainly complain of symptoms attributable to functional derangements of the proximal or the distal portions of the gut, while others (more numerous) present less-defined clinical expressions that are suggestive of an involvement of the whole gastrointestinal tract.

In recent years, technological improvements have led to the recognition of motor abnormalities, in many parts of the digestive canal, in the majority of patients affected by gastrointestinal functional syndromes (Fig. 4.4). Disrupted motility can be detected in the gastric antrum and proximal portions of the small bowel, in 50–60% of patients with ID, 70–80% of patients with associated IBS and ID, and in 100% of patients with CIIP. Disruptions of motor functions, therefore, appear to be more frequent in patients with more numerous and/or severe symptoms such as IBS+ID and CIIP patients. Nevertheless, gastroduodenal motor abnormalities are not specific: patients with prominent IBS symptoms present abnormal motor patterns similar to those of patients complaining

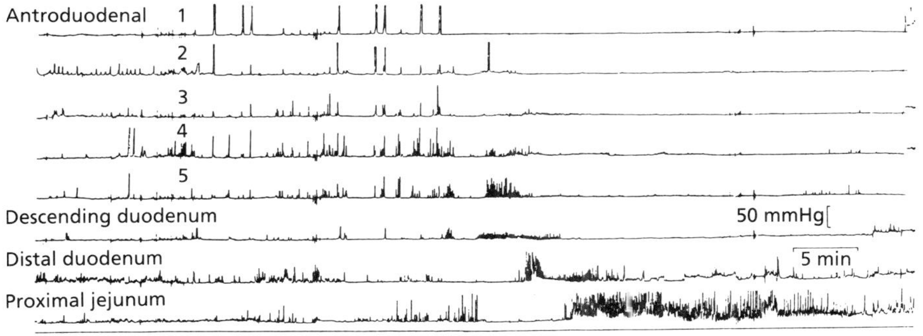

Fig. 4.4. Abnormal interdigestive migrating motor complex in a patient with unexplained abdominal pain, constipation and nausea (female, 20 years). Note the absence of phase I and of the antral component of phase III which presents an abnormal propagation in the proximal small bowel.

of prominent ID symptoms. These data seem to support the widely held opinion that gastrointestinal functional syndromes are different clinical expressions of common pathogenetic mechanisms (Read, 1987).

The actual role of motor factors in the pathogenesis of gastrointestinal functional syndromes remains to be defined. Studies designed to quantify the motor activities of the whole digestive canal in large groups of symptomatic and asymptomatic individuals are needed to clarify this intriguing problem. Some patients may have derangements of motor patterns that have not been adequately quantified, such as, in the proximal gut, the tonic pressure changes produced by the gastric fundus. Finally, digestive functions other than motility may be involved in the determination of certain symptoms.

Further studies need to be performed in this area, whose clinical relevance, probably underestimated for too long, is now fully recognized.

REFERENCES

Acharya, U., Waite, N., Howlett, P., Tanner, A.R. & Smith, C.L. (1983) Failure to demonstrate altered gastric emptying in irritable bowel syndrome. *Dig Dis Sci* **28**, 889–893.

Almy, T.P. (1983) Clinical features and diagnosis of functional GI disorders. In Chey, W.Y. (ed), *Functional Disorders of the Digestive Tract*, pp. 7–11. Raven Press, New York.

Barbara, L., Camilleri, M., Corinaldesi, R. *et al.* (1989) The definition and investigation of dyspepsia. Consensus of an *ad hoc* working party. *Dig Dis Sci* **34**, 1272–1276.

Bueno, L., Fioramonti, J., Ruckebush, Y., Frexinos, J. & Coulom, P. (1980) Evaluation of colonic myoelectrical activity in health and functional disorders. *Gut* **21**, 480–485.

Camilleri, M., Malagelada, J.R., Stanghellini, V., Fealey, R.D. & Sheps, S.G. (1985) Gastrointestinal motility disturbances in patients with orthostatic hypotension. *Gastroenterology* **88**, 1223–1231.

Camilleri, M., Malagelada, J.R., Kao, P.C. & Zinsmeister, A.R. (1986a) Gastric and autonomic responses to stress in functional dyspepsia. *Dig Dis Sci* **31**, 1169–1177.

Camilleri, M., Malagelada, J.R., Stanghellini, V., Zinsmeister, A.R., Kao, P.C. & Choh, H.L. (1986b) Dose related effects of synthetic human β-endorphin and naloxone on fed gastrointestinal motility. *Am J Physiol* **251**, G147–G154.

Colin-Jones, D.G., Bloom, B., Bodemar, G. *et al.* (1988) Management of dyspepsia: a report of a working party. *Lancet* **1**, 576–579.

Connel, A.M. (1962) The motility of the pelvic colon, II. Paradoxical motility in diarrhoea and constipation. *Gut* **3**, 342–348.

Feldman, M., Smith, H.J. & Simon, T.R. (1984) Gastric emptying of solid radio-opaque markers: studies in healthy subjects and diabetic patients. *Gastroenterology* **87**, 895–902.

Harrison, T.R. (1987) *Principles of Internal Medicine*, 10th edn. McGraw-Hill Book Co., New York.

Kellow, J.E. & Phillips, S.F. (1987) Altered small bowel motility in irritable bowel syndrome is correlated with symptoms. *Gastroenterology* **92**, 1885–1893.

Kellow, J.E., Phillips, S.F., Miller, L.J. & Zinsmeister, A.R. (1988) Dysmotility of the small intestine in irritable bowel syndrome. *Gut* **29**, 1236–1241.

Kruis W., Thieme, C.H., Weinzierl, M., Schussler, P., Holl, J. & Paulus, W. (1984) A diagnostic score for the irritable bowel syndrome. *Gastroenterology* 87, 1–7.

Kumar, D. & Wingate, D.L. (1985) The irritable bowel syndrome: a paroxysmal disorder. *Lancet* 2, 973–977.

Labò, G., Bortolotti, M., Vezzadini, P., Bonora, G. & Bersani, G. (1986) Interdigestive gastroduodenal motility and serum motilin levels in patients with idiopathic delay in gastric emptying. *Gastroenterology* 90, 20–26.

Lagarde, S.P. & Spiro, H.M. (1984) Non-ulcer dyspepsia. *Clinics Gastroenterol* 13, 437–446.

Latimer, P., Sarna, S., Campbell, D., Latimer, M., Waterfall, W. & Daniel, E.E. (1981) Colonic motor and myoelectric activity: a comparative study of normal subjects, psychoneurotic patients and patients with irritable bowel syndrome. *Gastroenterology* 80, 893–901.

Malagelada, J.R. & Camilleri, M. (1985) Disorders of the motility of the stomach. In Berk, J.E. (ed), *Bockus Gastroenterology*, pp. 1305–1327. W.B. Saunders, Philadelphia.

Malagelada, J.R. & Stanghellini, V. (1985) Manometric evaluation of functional upper gut symptoms. *Gastroenterology* 88, 1223–1231.

Malagelada, J.R., Camilleri, M. & Stanghellini, V. (1986) *Manometric Diagnosis of Gastrointestinal Motility Disorders*, 1st edn. Thieme, New York.

Maldonado, J.E., Gregg, J.A., Green, P.A. & Brown, A.L. (1970) Chronic idiopathic intestinal pseudo-obstruction. *Am J Med* 49, 203–212.

Manning, A.P., Thompson, W.G., Keaton, K.W. & Morris, A.F. (1978) Towards positive diagnosis of the irritable bowel. *Br Med J* 2, 653–654.

Read, N.W. (1987) Functional gastroenterological disorders: the name's the thing. *Gut* 28, 1–4.

Rees, W.D.W., Miller, L.J. & Malagelada, J.R. (1980) Dyspepsia, antral motor dysfunction, and gastric stasis of solids. *Gastroenterology* 78, 360–365.

Rhind, J.A. & Watson, L. (1968) Gallstone dyspepsia. *Br Med J* 1, 32.

Smart, H.L., Nicholson, D.A. & Atkinson, M. (1986) Gastro-oesophageal reflux in the irritable bowel syndrome. *Gut* 27, 1127–1131.

Snape, W.J. Jr, Carlson, G.M. & Cohen, S. (1976) Colonic myoectrical activity in the irritable bowel syndrome. *Gastroenterology* 70, 326–330.

Snape, W.J. Jr, Carlson, G.M. & Matarrazzo, S.A. (1977) Evidence that abnormal myoelectrical activity produces colonic motor dysfunction in the irritable bowel syndrome. *Gastroenterology* 70, 383–387.

Stanghellini, V., Malagelada, J.R., Zinsmeister, A.R., Go, V.L.W. & Kao, P.C. (1983) Stress-induced motor disturbances in humans: possible humoral mechanisms. *Gastroenterology* 85, 83–91.

Stanghellini, V., Malagelada, J.R., Zinsmeister, A.R., Go, V.L.W. & Kao, P.C. (1984) Effect of opiate and adrenergic blockers on the gut motor response to centrally acting stimuli. *Gastroenterology* 87, 1104–1113.

Stanghellini, V., Camilleri, M. & Malagelada, J.R. (1987) Chronic idiopathic intestinal pseudo-obstruction: clinical and intestinal manometric findings. *Gut* 28, 5–12.

Stanghellini, V., Corinaldesi, R. & Barbara, L. (1988a) Pseudo-obstruction syndromes. In Read, N.W. & Grundy, D. (eds), *Baillière's Clinical Gastroenterology 2. Gastrointestinal Neurophysiology*, pp. 225–254. Baillière Tindall, London.

Stanghellini, V., Corinaldesi, R., Salgemini, R. *et al.* (1988b) Gastric acid secretion and gastric emptying of solid and homogenized meals in patients with dyspeptic symptoms. *Gastroenterology* (abstr) 94, 441.

Sullivan, M.A., Cohen, S. & Snape, W.J. (1978) Colonic myoelectrical activity in irritable bowel syndrome: effect of eating and anticholinergics. *New Engl J Med* 298, 878–883.

Summers, R.W., Yanda, R., Prihoda, M. & Flatt, A. (1983) Acute intestinal obstruction: an electromyographic study in dogs. *Gastroenterology* 85, 1301–1306.

Talley, N.J. & Piper, D.W. (1986) Major life event stress and dyspepsia of unknown cause: a case control study. *Gut* 27, 127–134.

Taylor, I., Darby, C. & Hammond, P. (1978) Comparison of rectosigmoid myoelectrical activity in the irritable colon syndrome during relapses and remissions. *Gut* **19**, 923–929.

Telander, R.L., Morgan, K.G., Kreulen, D.L., Schmalz, P.F., Kelly, K.A. & Szurzewsky, J.H. (1978) Human gastric atony with tachygastria and gastric retention. *Gastroenterology* **75**, 497–501.

Thompson, D.G., Richelson, E. & Malagelada, J.R. (1982) Perturbation of gastric emptying and duodenal motility via the central nervous system. *Gastroenterology* **83**, 1200–1206.

Thompson, W.G. (1984) Non-ulcer dyspepsia. *Can Med Assoc J* 1, 330, 565–569.

Whorwell, P.J., Clouter, C. & Smith, C.L. (1981) Oesophageal motility in the irritable bowel syndrome. *Br Med J* **282**, 1101–1102.

Whorwell, P.J., Lupton, E.W., Erduran, D. & Wilson, K. (1986a) Bladder smooth muscle dysfunction in patients with irritable bowel syndrome. *Gut* **27**, 1014–1017.

Whorwell, P.J., McCallum, M., Creed, F.H. & Roberts, T. (1986b) Non-colonic features of irritable bowel syndrome. *Gut* **27**, 37–40.

Wood, J.D. (1973) Electrical activity of the intestine of mice with hereditary megacolon and absence of enteric ganglion cells. *Am J Dig Dis* **18**, 477–488.

You, O.H., Lee, K.Y., Chey, W.Y. & Menguy, R. (1980) Electrogastrographic study of patients with unexplained nausea, bloating and vomiting. *Gastroenterology* **79**, 311–314.

You, O.H., Chey W.Y., Lee, K.Y., Menguy, R. & Bartoff, A. (1981) Gastric and small intestinal myoelectric dysrhythmia associated with chronic intractable nausea and vomiting. *Ann Int Med* **95**, 449–451.

5 Extraintestinal Manifestations of the Irritable Bowel Syndrome

P.J. Whorwell

INTRODUCTION

The more symptoms of which a patient complains, the more suspicious a doctor becomes about the reality of that person's disease. Patients with irritable bowel syndrome (IBS) usually complain of abdominal pain, abdominal distension and an abnormal bowel habit. In addition, with increasing evidence of a more diffuse involvement of the gastrointestinal tract (Whorwell *et al.*, 1981; Kellow & Phillips, 1987), it is not surprising that patients also have other gastrointestinal symptoms depending on the localization of the abnormality. Thus, upper gastrointestinal complaints are also quite common in this disorder, leading to such diagnoses as reflux oesophagitis, non-ulcer dyspepsia and biliary dyskinesia. All this leads to a mounting list of symptoms for which extensive investigation is largely unrewarding. When the patient is then told there is nothing wrong, the patient becomes disillusioned with the doctor and the doctor starts to feel the patient is a chronic complainer. Once the doctor−patient relationship becomes compromised by this state of affairs, the patient is reluctant to admit to further symptomatology and keeps complaints to a minimum and certainly confined to the gastrointestinal system.

Some years ago we formed the clinical impression that patients with IBS were suffering from a series of non-colonic symptoms of which they were reluctant to complain. It was therefore decided to assess the more diffuse symptomatology of IBS and compare the prevalence of certain symptoms in 100 patients and 100 healthy controls (Whorwell *et al.*, 1986b). Table 5.1 lists those gastrointestinal symptoms and Table 5.2 those non-gastrointestinal symptoms which were significantly ($P < 0.001$) more common in IBS subjects. There is undoubtedly a raised incidence of psychopathology in patients with IBS (Creed & Guthrie, 1987) and it could be argued that this may account for some of these findings. For this reason patients were therefore divided into those with and without possible psychiatric disorder. There was no difference between the two groups in the prevalence of the symptoms listed in

Table 5.1. Gastrointestinal symptoms in patients with IBS ($P < 0.001$ compared with controls)

Symptom	Prevalence in IBS (%)	Prevalence in controls (%)
Nausea	29	2
Dysphagia	19	0
Early satiety	60	8
Dyspepsia	36	9
Excessive flatus	85	42

Table 5.2. Extraintestinal symptoms in patients with IBS ($P < 0.001$ compared with controls)

Symptom	Prevalence in IBS (%)	Prevalence in controls (%)
Back pain	68	28
Constant tiredness/lethargy	70	20
Bad breath/unpleasant taste in mouth	65	16
Frequent headaches	34	3
Urinary frequency	52	12
Urinary urgency	41	9
Nocturia	48	17
Incomplete emptying of bladder	50	18
Dyspareunia	41	5
Thigh pain	40	5

Table 5.2, although some psychological symptoms such as panic attacks and tremulousness were much less prominent in patients without psychiatric problems.

The presence of all these complaints in subjects with IBS, particularly those of an extraintestinal nature, raises many issues such as questions about their causation and the possibility of inappropriate investigation. Backache, thigh pain and profound lethargy are particularly difficult to account for, although they are very common. Lethargy is a frequent accompaniment of affective disorders, but in our study was no less common in subjects without any demonstrable psychopathology.

UROLOGICAL ABNORMALITIES

If IBS is a more diffuse disorder of smooth muscle than previously recognized, it is possible that smooth muscle outside the gastrointestinal system may be similarly affected. In view of the frequent finding of urological symptoms in these patients, we undertook urodynamic investigation of 30 subjects with IBS, comparing the findings to those of a control group of patients attending for

Table 5.3. Urodynamic findings in patients with IBS and controls

	IBS (%)	Controls (%)	IBS with urinary symtpoms (%)
Unstable bladder	33	3	100
Steep cystometrogram	17	10	80
Stable bladder	50	87	66

urodynamic assessment (Whorwell *et al.*, 1986a). These were patients with urinary symptoms referred to a urological clinic, but in whom there was no evidence of IBS. It was considered unethical to perform urodynamic measurements in normal controls, but as the control group selected already had urinary symptoms they would, if anything, be more likely to have abnormal results and bias against a positive finding in the IBS group. Fifty percent of the patients with IBS, compared to only 13% of controls ($P = 0.006$), had some demonstrable abnormality of bladder function (Table 5.3). Detrusor instability was observed in 33% of patients, compared with 3% of controls, and a steep cystometrogram was observed in 17% of patients compared with 10% of controls. Detrusor instability is defined as the occurrence of detrusor contractions which occur during passive filling of the bladder, which the patient is unable to inhibit, and which is associated with such symptoms as frequency, nocturia and urgency. It is interesting to note that patients in our study with a tendency to a frequent bowel habit were more likely to exhibit a detrusor instability. Thus, it appears that some patients with IBS have a demonstrable disorder of bladder smooth muscle or its innervation, and it is tempting to speculate that this may be in some way associated with the pathophysiological process underlying IBS.

GYNAECOLOGICAL ABNORMALITIES

As can be seen from Table 5.2, dyspareunia is common in women with IBS and this led us to speculate that there might be an adverse effect on sexual function. Fifty females with IBS were studied and 30 patients with colonic inflammatory bowel disease; 30 patients with duodenal ulceration served as controls (Guthrie *et al.*, 1987). All subjects were interviewed by a female psychiatrist in the privacy of their own home. Eighty-three percent of IBS patients admitted to sexual dysfunction which they attributed to their gastrointestinal disorder (Table 5.4). The comparative figures for the inflammatory bowel disease and peptic ulcer patients were 30% and 16% respectively ($P < 0.001$). There was little change in the results when the data were re-analysed excluding patients with psychiatric disorder.

Table 5.4. Sexual function in women with irritable bowel syndrome (IBS), inflammatory bowel disease (IBD), and duodenal ulceration (DU)

	IBS (%)	IBD (%)	DU (%)
Sexual function adversely affected by gastrointestinal disorder	83	30	16
Abdominal pain on sexual intercourse	69	7	0
Vaginal pain on sexual intercourse	17	7	12

By far the commonest complaint was the provocation, by sexual intercourse, of a pain similar to that associated with IBS and characteristically the onset of the pain was often delayed by several hours. It is not clear whether the pain arises from smooth muscle or not and if it does, whether it is gastrointestinal or genital tract in origin. However, its similarity to IBS pain suggests it may originate from the bowel. This is an aspect of IBS which would not be routinely enquired after in a gastroenterology clinic, but is probably of considerable practical importance. Such a problem could well induce marital disharmony and the stress associated with this may well lead to an exacerbation of the IBS.

The gynaecological aspects of IBS have received little attention and we have recently taken an interest in them. Preliminary data from our unit suggests that IBS is very common in patients attending gynaecological clinics, particularly in those referred for abdominal pain. In addition we have found that the outcome of a gynaecological consultation is significantly less satisfactory if symptoms suggestive of IBS are present (Prior & Whorwell, 1989a; Prior *et al.*, 1989).

CONCLUSIONS

The multiplicity of symptoms in IBS may lead to referral to many different specialties, depending on which predominate. Thus urologists, gynaecologists and even orthopaedic surgeons may become involved in management. A series of inappropriate investigations, occasionally leading to unnecessary surgery, may follow all to no avail. Patients are often greatly relieved to find a medical practitioner who recognizes that their seemingly unrelated symptoms can be attributed to IBS. Capacity to cope with these extraintestinal manifestations of IBS is often dramatically improved even if treatment does little to alleviate them.

REFERENCES

Creed, F.H. & Guthrie, E. (1987) Psychological factors in the irritable bowel syndrome. *Gut* 28, 1307–1318.

Guthrie, E., Creed, F.H. & Whorwell, P.J. (1987) Severe sexual dysfunction in females with irritable syndrome: a comparison with inflammatory bowel disease and peptic ulceration. *Br Med J* 295, 577–578.

Kellow, J.E. & Phillips, S.F. (1987) Altered small bowel motility in irritable bowel syndrome is correlated wth symptoms. *Gastroenterology* 92, 1885–1893.

Prior, A. & Whorwell, P.J. (1989) Gynaecological consultations in patients with irritable bowel syndrome. *Gut* 30, 996–998.

Prior, A., Wilson, K., Whorwell, P.J. & Fanagher, E.B. (1989) Irritable bowel syndrome in the gynaecological clinic: a survey of 798 new referrals. *Dig Dis Sci* 34, 1820–1824.

Whorwell, P.J., Clouter, C. & Smith, C.L. (1981) Oesophageal motility in the irritable bowel syndrome. *Br Med J* 282, 1101–1102.

Whorwell, P.J., Lupton, E.W., Erduran, D. & Wilson, K. (1986a) Bladder smooth muscle abnormalities in patients with irritable bowel syndrome. *Gut* 27, 1014–1017.

Whorwell, P.J., McCallum, M., Creed, F.H. & Roberts, C.T. (1986b) Non-colonic features of irritable bowel syndrome. *Gut* 27, 37–40.

Section 3
Autonomic Nerves, Stress and Hypnosis

6 Involvement of Extrinsic Nerves in Functional Disorders of the Bowel

D. Grundy

INTRODUCTION

Irritable bowel syndrome (IBS) is a common complaint whose diagnosis is largely based on symptoms for which no obvious cause can be found. Indeed, it is estimated that as many as 30% of the general population suffer from IBS without seeking medical advice (Thomson & Heaton, 1980). This raises the question 'what is normal?' with regards sensations emanating from the bowel and 'what causes an individual to seek medical help?'—questions which have led to the suggestion that IBS may be the result of an abnormal perception of normal gut activity (Drossman & Sancler, 1985). The link between psychiatric disorders and IBS is used to substantiate the argument that it is a disease of the mind and not a gastro-enterological complaint (Liss *et al.*, 1973; Young *et al.*, 1976). However, because of the delicate perceptions of the central nervous system (CNS) and the varied emotional states that ensue, such things as stress and anxiety, and charged emotions like anger and fear, can have profound effects on the gastrointestinal tract. Irritable bowel syndrome may therefore be the outward signs of autonomic dysfunction undetectable with present clinical diagnostic techniques. Indeed, because of the complexity of the enteric and autonomic control mechanisms revealed by recent developments in neuro-physiology and neurochemistry, it is quite conceivable that subtle changes within these reflex pathways could have profound effects on gastrointestinal function. In this chapter I intend to extrapolate from our current knowledge of extrinsic neural control mechanisms (especially relating to the vagal innervation) in order to discuss the possible ways in which inappropriate neural activity may give rise to IBS. By necessity this involves considerable speculation.

As a starting point I have outlined a working definition of IBS. This is in no way meant to be conclusive, but merely provides a basis from which to gauge neural involvement.

1 IBS is a functional disorder of the gastrointestinal tract (especially musculature) which can affect its entire length and accessory organs.

2 It can be triggered or exacerbated either from the CNS (i.e.

stress) or from within the gut lumen (i.e. food allergy, gastro-enteritis) (Cann & Read, 1985; Kumar & Wingate, 1985).

3 It is associated with hyperresponsiveness of the effector (muscle) as indicated, for example, by an increased sensitivity of the rectum to rectal distension, bile salts, cholecystokinin (CCK) (Flynn *et al.*, 1981; Harvey & Read, 1973; Ritchie, 1973). A recent paper by Kellow *et al.* (1988) indicates that this hyperresponsiveness extends into the small bowel. However, hyperreactivity does not necessarily translate into hyperactivity. If the level of activity *per se* was the determining factor, then one must question why the activity front of the interdigestive migrating motor complex, or the migrating bursts of colonic contractions, do not normally give rise to the symptomatic complaints of the IBS sufferer. It is what the contractions do in terms of the luminal contents that is more likely to be important and this depends on the coordination of adjacent segments of bowel.

4 Symptoms are associated with hyperreactivity in one or more regions of the gastrointestinal tract (commonly colon). Since these tend to occur intermittently it makes the clinical study of the underlying causes of IBS difficult.

Extrinsic nerves and the 'normal' gut

Since the complex question of visceral sensitivity is covered in Chapter 9, I will concentrate on the interactions between the extrinsic and the enteric nervous mechanisms controlling gastrointestinal function. However, because the extrinsic autonomic innervation is predominantly afferent (Grundy, 1988a) conveying information from the wall and lumen of the bowel, quite apart from that encoding noxious events, I must touch on the role of this afferent supply in generating extrinsic neural reflexes.

Activity in the parasympathetic and sympathetic preganglionic neurones supplying the gastrointestinal tract is generated within the CNS, but modified according to the enormous amount of afferent information reaching the brainstem and spinal cord from the abdominal viscera. Information is relayed centrally in afferent fibres, whose properties are determined by the location of the receptor endings within the gut wall. Thus, receptors in the mucosa are sensitive to the physical and chemical nature of luminal contents, while others in the muscle layer behave as in-series tension receptors responding to both distension and contractions of the bowel wall. Other receptors following a predominantly splanchnic pathway have endings in the serosal and mesenteric connections and respond to distortion of the viscera. This highly convergent afferent input, through reflex pathways in the spinal cord and brainstem, sets the appropriate level of discharge in the autonomic outflow to the gut. In other words, the level of neuronal activity in the autonomic supply to the gut is determined by the nature of the afferent information it receives. The afferent information is integrated within the brainstem and spinal cord, and the net outcome is a particular pattern and frequency of action potentials in the various preganglionic parasympathetic and sympathetic neurones (Grundy, 1988b; Janig, 1988; Morrison, 1988). These action potentials therefore carry the coded message to the gastrointestinal tract, which serves to coordinate the activity in regions of the bowel up to several metres apart, and adjust the various motor, secretory and possibly absorptive functions to the overall needs of digestion. One tends to think of reflexes through these pathways being switched on by appropriate stimuli, and in the absence of these stimuli the pathways are switched off. However, because the incoming afferent signals are integrated with information generated centrally, individual efferent neurones can show a spectrum of response ranging from inhibition or complete suppression of ongoing activity to powerful excitation (Davison & Grundy, 1978; Grundy *et al.*, 1981; Blackshaw *et al.*, 1987).

This capacity for both inhibition and excitation adds another dimension to the control process, since besides the possibility of relaxation resulting from the activation of inhibitory pathways, or contraction occurring due to activation of excitatory pathways, one can achieve the same motor event by disinhibition of the appropriate motor pathway. Indeed, for the vagus nerve it has been suggested that there is reciprocal modulation of the excitatory and inhibitory pathways (Davison & Grundy, 1978).

The activity in the excitatory and inhibitory autonomic nerves has widespread influences on the gastrointestinal tract (Grundy, 1988b), but, the importance of this extrinsic influence is often questioned because of the relative paucity of efferent neurones in the extrinsic supply compared to the enteric nervous system (ENS). The ENS with its millions of neurones functions as a 'gut-brain'. It can function independently from the extrinsic supply and contains the hard-wired circuits that regulate the various gastrointestinal functions. Thus the concept of 'command neurones' in the ENS is rapidly gaining credibility. All that may be required of the extrinsic supply is to modulate these hard-wired motor programmes. Consistent with this suggestion is the observation that, in addition to the preganglionic parasympathetic input to the ENS, much of the postganglionic sympathetic innervation also terminates around the enteric ganglia and may modulate transmission through reflex pathways in the ENS (Furness & Costa, 1987).

The power of the extrinsic supply is readily demonstrated in acute experiments when the extrinsic nerves are electrically stimulated or sectioned. However, chronic denervation causes only temporary disruption of gastrointestinal functions, because of plasticity within the enteric supply which can adapt to the loss of extrinsic input. Under normal circumstances, however, the extrinsic influences can modulate the sensitivity of the gut to both local refexes and circulating hormones. One example of this 'permissive role' for the extrinsic nerves is the reflex increase in antral motility observed during antral distension. This is potentiated by a vagal efferent input but not dependent as such on a vagal reflex; an afferent input to the brainstem is not required except to set the appropriate level of tonic discharge in the efferent fibres (Grundy *et al.*, 1986). In this way the extrinsic supply may 'gate' reflexes mediated through the ENS and also responses to local and systemic humoral agents. One can envisage in the two extremes the gates being open or shut. However, regulating the degree to which these are 'ajar' gives fine control of effector activity. The gates may also operate in the opposite direction with local neural and hormonal effects modulating the sensitivity to extrinsic influences.

Extrinsic nerves and the gut in irritable bowel syndrome

Under normal circumstances there is a hierarchy of controls regulating gastrointestinal functions with two main levels at which integration takes place. Within the brainstem and spinal cord there are reflex circuits which determine the extent to which incoming afferent activity gives rise to an appropriate level of discharge in the excitatory and inhibitory efferent pathways. These reflexes are regulated from higher brain regions. Within the ENS local reflexes control effector responses and are modulated by extrinsic, enteric and hormonal controls. One can visualize how a dysfunction at either of these sites could modify the sensitivity to luminal stimuli and extrinsic neural and humoral inputs, which would therefore respond inappropriately to what might otherwise be normal stimuli. Inappropriate responses would lead to the abnormal motor activity reported in IBS patients and by disturbing the flow of digesta give rise to the symptomatic complaints.

Hyperresponsiveness of the gastrointestinal tract could arise through descending influences from higher brain regions as a consequence of emotional stress or anxiety. Such descending influences would modify the transmission through the extrinsic reflex centres in the brainstem and spinal cord and give rise to altered levels of activity in the preganglionic neurones. This in turn would alter the sensitivity of the gastrointestinal tract to local reflexes through the ENS or the circulating hormones, giving rise to inappropriate responses, abnormal motor activity and the IBS condition. The outcome would be the same if the activity in the extrinsic supply remained normal but the ENS became more sensitive to this existing activity. This could occur through subtle changes in transmitter output or the density of pre- or postsynaptic receptors within the ENS. This would inevitably change the level of excitability of neurones in the ENS, disturbing the delicate balance between excitatory and inhibitory inputs and taking the neurone nearer to threshold for activation, be it through local or extrinsic reflex pathways.

The primary defect need not necessarily arise in the integrative circuitry. The same inappropriate response might also arise from a change in the sensitivity of afferent endings within the gut wall in a way analagous to changes in the airways during asthma. Inappropriate afferent discharge could, through reflex pathways in the brainstem and spinal cord, result in inappropriate levels of discharge in the extrinsic efferent supply or, through enteric reflexes, increase the sensitivity of the ENS to descending influences in the autonomic nerves or to hormones. The net effect of either would be the augmentation of reflex activity leading to inappropriate responses and the IBS condition.

The way in which afferent endings may become sensitized is unclear, but it could involve the erosion of the mucosal barrier which normally buffers the epithelium layer from the luminal contents. Another possibility could be as a consequence of the afferent terminations being sensitive to endogenous paracrine or endocrine substances (see Chapter 10).

CONCLUSIONS

Several possible ways in which extrinsic nerves may interact with the ENS to cause hyperreactivity of the bowel leading to IBS are presented. In Fig. 6.1 the way in which these different sites interact

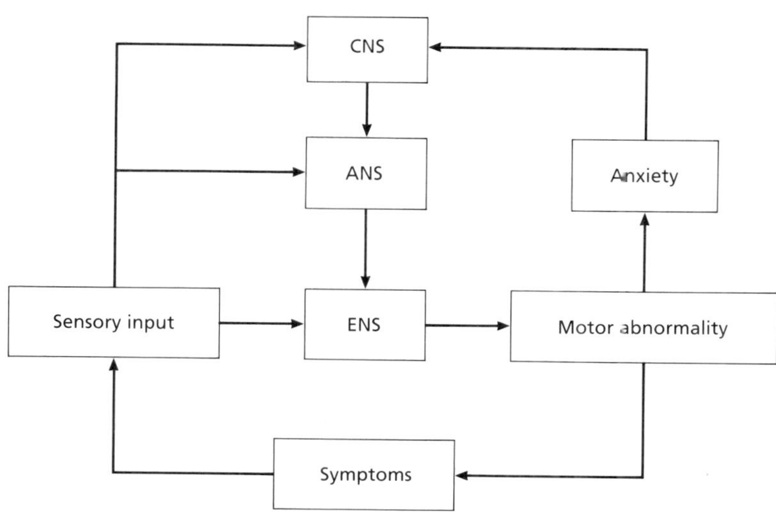

Fig. 6.1. Systems model of the interactions between intrinsic and extrinsic neural pathways in the genesis of IBS. (ANS = autonomic nervous system; CNS = central nervous system; ENS = enteric nervous system.)

is shown diagramatically. One can envisage a loop whereby exaggerated autonomic reflexes would result in the bowel responding inappropriately to otherwise normal stimuli which, through the symptoms thus caused, maintain the exaggerated autonomic outflow. In addition, the afferent inflow arising because of motor abnormalities will itself be reflected, through reflex connections in the brainstem and spinal cord, in a discordant autonomic outflow. Any treatment which breaks this loop would be effective and may explain the success of such diverse treatments as diet, hypnotherapy, antispasmodics and tranquillizers in the management of IBS.

REFERENCES

Blackshaw, L.A., Grundy, D. & Scratcherd, T. (1987) Involvement of gastrointestinal mechano- and intestinal chemoreceptors in vagal reflexes: an electrophysiological study. *J Auton Nerv Syst* **18**, 225–234.

Cann, P.A. & Read, N.W. (1985) A disease of the whole gut. In Read N.W. (ed), *Irritable Bowel Syndrome*, pp. 53–60. Grune & Stratton, London.

Davison, J.S. & Grundy, D. (1978) Modulation of single vagal efferent fibre discharge by gastrointestinal afferents in the rat. *J Physiol* **284**, 69–82.

Drossman, D.A. & Sandler, R.S. (1985) Irritable bowel syndrome: The role of psychosocial factors. In Read N.W. (ed), *Irritable Bowel Syndrome*, pp. 67–74. Grune & Stratton, London.

Flynn, M., Hammond, P., Darby, C., Hyland, J. & Taylor, I. (1981) Faecal bile acids and the irritable bowel syndrome. *Digestion* **22**, 144–149.

Furness, J.B. & Costa, M. (1987) *The Enteric Nervous System*, pp. 290. Churchill Livingstone, Melbourne.

Grundy, D. (1988a) Speculations of the structure/function relationship for vagal and splanchnic afferent endings supplying the gastrointestinal tract. *J Auton Nerv Syst* **22**, 175–180.

Grundy, D. (1988b) Vagal control of gastrointestinal function. In Read, N.J. & Grundy, D. (eds), *Baillière's Clinical Gastroenterology 2 (1)*, pp. 23–43. Baillière Tindall, London.

Grundy, D., Salih, A.A. & Scratcherd T. (1981) Modulation of vagal efferent discharge by mechanoreceptors in the stomach, duodenum and colon of the ferret. *J Physiol* **319**, 43–52.

Grundy, D., Hutson, D. & Scratcherd, T (1986) A permissive role for the vagus nerves in the genesis of antro-antral reflexes in the anaesthetized ferret. *J Physiol* **381**, 377–384.

Harvey, R.F. & Read, A.E. (1973) Effect of cholecystokinin on colonic motility and symptoms in patients with the irritable bowel syndrome. *Lancet* **i**, 7791–3.

Jänig, W. (1988) Integration of gut function by sampalletin reflexes. In Read, N.J. & Grundy, D. (eds), *Baillière's Clinical Gastroenterology 2 (1)*, pp. 45–62. Baillière Tindall, London.

Kellow, J.E., Phillips, S.F., Miller, L.J. & Zinsmeister, A.R. (1988) Dysmotility of the small intestine in irritable bowel syndrome. *Gut* **29**, 1236–1243.

Kumar, D. & Wingate, D.L. (1985) The IBS. A paroxysmal motor disorder. *Lancet* **ii**, 973–977.

Liss, J.L., Alpers, D. & Woodruff, R.A. (1973) The irritable colon syndrome and psychiatric illness. *Dis Nerv Syst* **34**, 151–157.

Morrison, J.F.B. (1988) The neural control of pelvic viscera. In Read, N.J. & Grundy, D. (eds), *Baillière's Clinical Gastroenterology 2 (1)*, pp. 63–84. Baillière Tindall, London.

Ritchie, J. (1973) Pain from distension of the pelvic colon by inflating a balloon in the irritable bowel syndrome. *Gut* **6**, 105–112.

Thompson, W.G. & Heaton, K.W. (1980) Functional bowel disorders in apparently healthy people. *Gastroenterology* **79**, 283–288.

Young, J.J., Alpers, D.H., Norland, C.C. & Woodruff, R.A. (1976) Psychiatric illness of the IBS: practical implications for the primary physician. *Gastroenterology* **70**, 162–166.

7 *A Study of Vagal Function in the Irritable Bowel Syndrome*

H.L. Smart

INTRODUCTION

The irritable bowel syndrome (IBS) is a common gastrointestinal disorder (Thompson & Heaton, 1980) which is frequently associated with oesophageal symptoms. Sixty years ago Bockus found that 'nausea, vomiting, pyrosis, anorexia, regurgitation and so-called biliousness' were frequent accompaniments of this condition (Bockus *et al.*, 1928). Recent studies have confirmed his original finding that symptoms referrable to the oesophagus occur in up to half of all IBS patients (Watson *et al.*, 1976, 1978; Rubin *et al.*, 1979; Dotevall *et al.*, 1982; Smart *et al.*, 1986; Whorwell *et al.*, 1986).

The major symptom complex would appear to be that of gastro-oesophageal reflux (GOR) (Rubin *et al.*, 1979; Dotevall *et al.*, 1982; Smart *et al.*, 1986): although globus sensation and dysphagia are not uncommon (Watson *et al.*, 1978; Smart *et al.*, 1986; Whorwell *et al.*, 1986). Investigation of the oesophageal abnormality in IBS has been limited. Although oesophageal dysmotility has been found (Watson *et al.*, 1976), the most consistent abnormality appears to be a hypotensive lower oesophageal sphincter (Whorwell *et al.*, 1981; Smart *et al.*, 1986). This is associated with pathological GOR (detected on oesophageal pH monitoring) in 50% of cases and macroscopic oesophagitis in over one-third (Smart *et al.*, 1986).

Symptomatic GOR is itself a common condition, with up to 36% of apparently healthy people having heartburn, acid regurgitation or both once a month or more often (Nebel *et al.*, 1976). Why this condition frequently coexists with IBS is unknown. Gastro-oesophageal reflux occurs as a result of failure of the antireflux mechanism, the principal component of which is the lower oesophageal sphincter. The resting tone of the sphincter unfortunately fails to differentiate adequately between normals and those with GOR (Atkinson *et al.*, 1957; MacLaurin, 1963), although the mean resting sphincter pressure tends to be lower in patients with oesophagitis (Dodds *et al.*, 1975a). In normal subjects, the pressure in the lower oesophageal sphincter rises with increasing intra-abdominal pressure (Ogilvie & Atkinson, 1984). This rise is abolished by truncal vagotomy and atropine suggesting that sphincter competence depends on a cholinergic mechanism mediated by a vagovagal reflex arc (Ogilvie & Atkinson, 1984).

This protective response is impaired in the majority of patients with reflux oesophagitis (Ogilvie *et al.*, 1985) in whom other evidence of vagal dysfunction also exists—abnormal gastric secretory responses to insulin/pentagastrin and disordered cardiac vagal reflexes (Heatley *et al.*, 1980; Ogilvie *et al.*, 1985). In this context, investigation of vagal function in patients with IBS might shed light on the association of GOR with this condition. The methods, results and implications of such an investigation are described in the following article.

PATIENTS AND METHODS

Twenty-five consecutive patients attending a gastroenterology clinic with IBS were studied. Their mean age was 39 years (range 24–61) and there were 15 women and 10 men. Patients were judged to have IBS if they complained of abdominal pain and disordered bowel habit of at least 1 year's duration. The symptoms described by Manning *et al.* (1978) as being common in IBS were used as positive indicators of the presence of this disorder. In 11 patients diarrhoea predominated, six had constipation, while the remainder had variable bowel habits. All patients had normal findings on clinical examination, sigmoidoscopy (with biopsy), stool culture and barium enema. Haematological and biochemical tests were all normal. The patients were unselected for the presence of oesophageal symptoms or predominant bowel habit. All were symptomatic (abdominal pain at least three times/week) at the time of their study and were not taking medication (especially anticholinergics) which could interfere with the test results.

Prior to the commencement of vagal function studies, all patients underwent detailed oesophageal investigation by endoscopy and biopsy, manometry and prolonged pH monitoring. The results of these studies are described in detail elsewhere (Smart *et al.*, 1986) and are summarized in Fig. 7.1.

Response of the lower oesophageal sphincter to increased intra-abdominal pressure

The study was performed in fasting subjects who had not taken medication for 48 hours beforehand. Intraluminal oesophageal and gastric pressures were measured with a triple-lumen polyvinyl catheter (external diameter 3.5 mm), which had three recording orifices equidistant from the tip and radially orientated at 120 degree intervals (Ogilvie & Atkinson, 1984). The catheter was

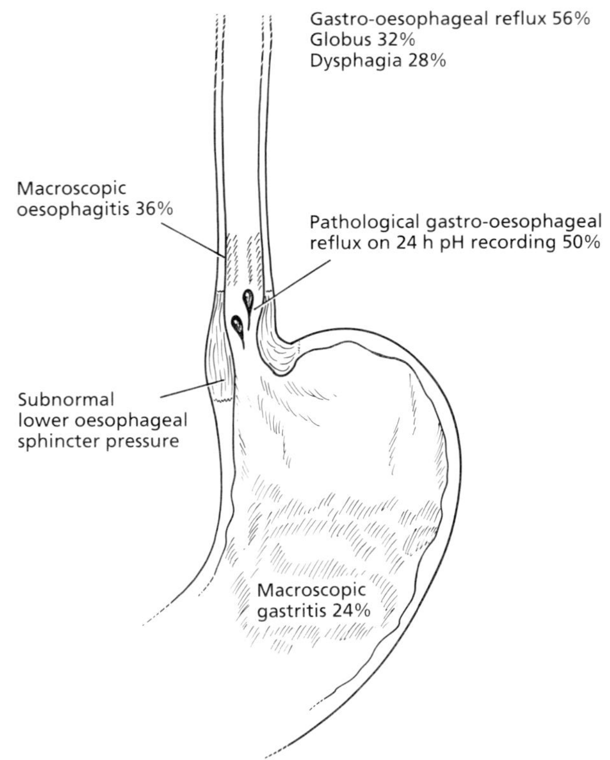

Fig. 7.1. The results of detailed oesophageal investigations in 25 patients with IBS (redrawn with permission from Smart *et al.*, 1986).

perfused constantly with distilled water at a rate of 0.6 ml/minute from a standard low-compliance hydraulic capillary infusion system (Model PIP-2, Mui Scientific, Ontario, Canada). Pressure changes were sensed by transducers (Gould P23 10, Gould Inc, Oxnard, California, USA), connected to an ink-writing polygraph (Model 7D, Grass Instruments, Quincy, Massachusetts, USA) onto which recordings were made.

The catheter was passed nasally into the stomach, the patient placed supine and rested for 15 minutes prior to the study. The position of the lower oesophageal sphincter was then identified using the station pull-through technique and its pressure recorded using the rapid pull-through technique of oesophageal manometry (Dodds *et al.*, 1975b). Five rapid pull-throughs were performed with the patient's breath held in expiration.

Intragastric pressure was taken as the difference between fundal pressure in expiration and atmospheric pressure. Lower oesophageal sphincter pressure was taken as the difference between maximum pressure recorded in the sphincter and the intragastric pressure, using the mean value obtained from the 15 pressure recordings.

After determining the basal lower oesophageal sphincter pressure, a thigh sphygmomanometer cuff mounted in a firm binder was passed around the patient's waist and fastened tightly. A moulded perspex plate in the pocket of the binder ensured that any increase in the cuff pressure was directed towards the abdominal wall rather than towards the binder. With the binder in position, the cuff was then inflated at increments of 10 mmHg until the patient experienced discomfort, usually around 50–60 mmHg. Five rapid pull-throughs were performed at each level of cuff pressure. Since intragastric pressure was not closely related to the pressure in the cuff, because of the variable resistance of the anterior abdominal wall, changes in lower oesophageal sphincter pressure were recorded in relation to changes in intragastric pressure as proposed by Ogilvie and Atkinson (1984).

A group of 25 age- and sex-matched subjects, free from symptoms of GOR and IBS, were used as controls in the assessment of the lower oesophageal sphincter's response to increased intra-abdominal pressure.

Gastric secretory responses

Patients were studied after an overnight fast. They were instructed not to smoke for 12 hours prior to the test and any medication likely to affect gastric acidity was stopped for at least 48 hours beforehand. A double-lumen salem-sump-type tube was passed into the stomach and its position checked with a water recovery test. Gastric secretions were then collected by continuous hand suction after insulin-induced hypoglycaemia and pentagastrin (Venables, 1970).

A phenol-red marker was used to correct for collection errors and pyloric losses (Hobsley & Silen, 1969) and electrolyte concentrations of the gastric juice were used to assess swallowed saliva and duodenogastric reflux (Faber *et al.*, 1974).

After a 30 minute basal collection period, sufficient soluble insulin (0.15 units/kg) was given intravenously to achieve a blood glucose concentration of 2.2 mmol/litre or less and gastric secretions were collected for 120 minutes in 15-minute fractions. Subsequently, pentagastrin (6 µg/kg) was given subcutaneously, and gastric secretions collected for a further 60 minutes.

The ratio of the peak acid output after insulin-induced hypoglycaemia, to the maximal acid output after pentagastrin, provides a measure of the intactness of gastric vagal innervation. Earlier investigations have shown this ratio to be greater than 0.7 in patients with untreated duodenal ulcer and consistently less than 0.7 after complete truncal vagotomy (Ogilvie & Atkinson, 1984). As it was considered unethical to perform insulin-pentagastrin tests on normal subjects, the results of patients with IBS were compared to those obtained in earlier work, from the same department, as detailed by Ogilvie (Ogilvie & Atkinson, 1984).

Heart rate variability with deep respiration

In resting man, the cyclical variation in heart rate with respiration is accentuated by deep breathing (Wheeler & Watkins, 1973) and is at maximum at six breaths per minute (Bennett *et al.*, 1978). To study this response, the patient, resting supine, was connected to a cardiac monitor (capable of detecting an immediate variation in heart rate) linked to a flat bed recorder. After a period of quiet respiration, the patient was instructed to breathe deeply in and out six times over a minute. The resulting variations in heart rate were recorded via the monitor onto the pen chart. For each breath the maximum and minimum heart rate was calculated and subtracted from each other. The mean difference from the six breaths was used as the heart rate variability. At the time of the study no patient was taking medication which would interfere with the heart rate variability.

Bennett has shown that normal subjects invariably have differences in heart rate of more than 15 beats per minute, with minimum levels varying with age: diabetics with autonomic neuropathy have differences of 10 beats per minute or less (Bennett *et al.*, 1978). Dr Bennett has been in the forefront of studying autonomic function in diabetes and has established a broad database of normal heart rate variation with age. I am grateful to him for allowing me to use those values for comparison with IBS patients.

Statistical analysis

Parametric data was analysed using a Student's *t*-test and non-parametric data by chi-square analysis, Fisher's exact probability test (2-sided) or the Mann–Whitney U test. Correlation between the results of the investigations was assessed by Spearman's rank correlation coefficient.

RESULTS

Response of the lower oesophageal sphincter to increased intra-abdominal pressure

Oesophageal manometry was tolerated by all IBS and control patients. Mean resting intragastric pressure and the mean change induced in intragastric pressure by abdominal compression were similar in both groups (Table 7.1). Although higher in control patients, the lower oesophageal sphincter pressure did not differ significantly from that of the IBS group. However, the response of

Table 7.1. Results of rapid pull-through oesophageal manometry in controls and IBS patients. Values are mean ± standard deviation in cmH_2O

	IBS	Controls
Resting intragastric pressure	6.4 ± 4.4	6.4 ± 4.7
Change in intragastric pressure with abdominal compression	9.4 ± 3.3	9.3 ± 4.1
Resting lower oesophageal sphincter pressure	19.0 ± 9.4	23.3 ± 10.1
Maximum change in lower oesophageal sphincter pressure with abdominal compression	1.9 ± 8.7	$7.1 \pm 4.5*$

* $P < 0.02$.

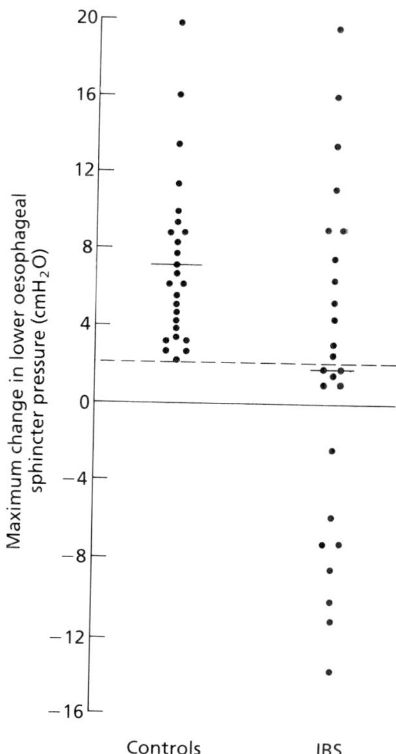

Fig. 7.2. The response of the lower oesophageal sphincter to elevation of intragastric pressure in controls and IBS patients. The broken line represents the lower limit of the normal response in the control subjects. The unbroken lines represent the mean maximum change in lower oesophageal sphincter pressure for each group of subjects.

the sphincter to abdominal compression was markedly different in the IBS patients and controls (Table 7.1).

With abdominal compression, for any given rise in intragastric pressure, all control subjects responded by increasing their lower oesophageal sphincter pressure by between 2 and 19.8 cmH$_2$O (Fig. 7.2). This finding was in keeping with that of Ogilvie and Atkinson (1984) who regard it as the most sensitive discriminant between normal and abnormal vagal function.

Elevation of intragastric pressure produced maximum changes in the level of lower oesophageal sphincter pressure from baseline of between -13.5 and 19.9 cmH$_2$O in patients with IBS. Only 12 of the 25 subjects studied showed a response above that of the lowest level seen in the control group (Fig. 7.2).

Gastric secretory responses

Gastric secretory studies were performed on 23 of the 25 patients with IBS, all of whom experienced symptomatic hypoglycaemia. Gastric secretory parameters obtained showed a peak acid output after insulin of 21.6 $\pm$ 13.6 mmol/hour (mean $\pm$ standard deviation) and a maximal acid output after pentagastrin of 27.6 $\pm$ 15.5 mmol/hour. Plotting the ratio of these two parameters to obtain an index of the intactness of vagal supply to the parietal cells of the stomach, and comparing the values obtained for IBS patients to those reported by Ogilvie and Atkinson (1984) working in the same laboratory with duodenal ulcer subjects, it can be seen that seven of the 23 patients studied yielded a subnormal result (Fig. 7.3), indicating impaired efferent vagal function.

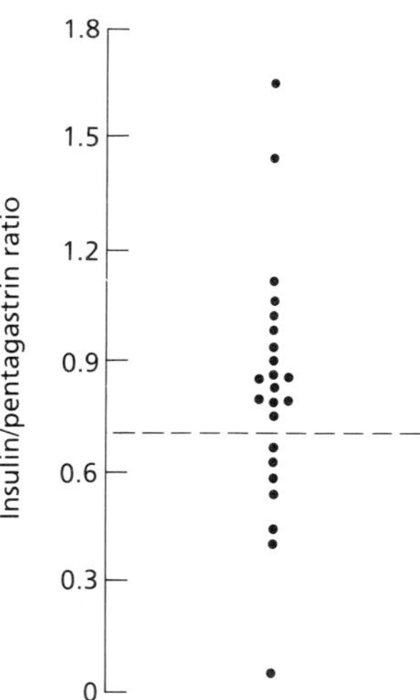

Fig. 7.3. The results of gastric secretory studies in patients with IBS. The broken line represents the lower limit of the normal response (redrawn with permission from Ogilvie & Atkinson, 1984).

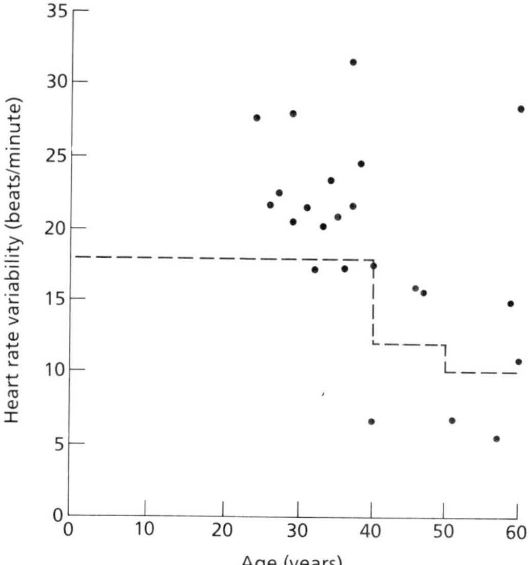

Fig. 7.4. The results of heart rate variability in patients with IBS. The broken line represents the lower limit of the normal response for a given age range.

Heart rate variability with deep respiration

In normal subjects heart rate variability shows a decline with increasing age. With allowance for age, six of 23 patients with IBS showed a subnormal heart rate variability with deep respiration (Fig. 7.4).

Relationship between tests of vagal function, patient characteristics and oesophageal abnormalities

Patients with abnormal vagal function tended to be older than those in whom vagal function was normal (Table 7.2). This difference however was not statistically significant. There was no obvious relationship between abnormal vagal function and the sex of the patient. Vagal dysfunction was more common in patients with a longer duration of IBS symptoms, with a significant difference being present ($P < 0.01$) when considering the response of the lower oesophageal sphincter to increased intra-abdominal pressure (Table 7.2). Abnormality of vagal function was unrelated to the bowel habit of the patient.

Abnormalities in either gastrointestinal or cardiac vagal function were not closely related to the presence or absence of GOR symptoms, macroscopic oesophageal disease, resting lower oesophageal sphincter pressure or the results of 24-hour distal oesophageal pH recording (Table 7.2).

Table 7.2. Tests of vagal function in relation to patient characteristics and oesophageal abnormality

	Lower oesophageal sphincter response to increased intra-abdominal pressure		Gastric secretory response		Heart rate variability	
	Normal*	Abnormal	Normal[†]	Abnormal	Normal[‡]	Abnormal
Number of patients (M, F)	12 (7, 5)	13 (3, 10)	16 (9, 7)	7 (1, 6)	17 (1, 16)	6 (2, 4)
Mean age (SD, years)	37.7 (10.5)	40.0 (12.0)	36.1 (6.5)	43.8 (16.1)	38.3 (12.1)	42.7 (4.5)
Median duration of IBS symptoms (range, years)	2 (1−6)	5 (2−11)	2 (1−7)	5 (1.5−8)	2 (1−6)	6 (1−11)
Symptoms of GOR						
× 1/month or more often	9	5	11	2	11	3
Less often	3	8	5	5	6	3
Macroscopic oesophageal disease	5	4	7	2	7	2
Mean resting lower oesophageal sphincter pressure (SD, cmH$_2$O)	15.0 (6.4)	13.0 (4.0)	13.6 (5.5)	13.8 (4.0)	14.6 (5.5)	13.5 (3.5)
24-hour pH monitoring						
Abnormal GOR	5	6	7	3	8	2
Normal	6	5	7	3	6	4

* 2 cmH$_2$O or more.
[†] Ratio 0.7 or more.
[‡] Between 18 and 8 beats/minute, dependent on age.
M = male. F = female. SD = standard deviation. GOR = gastro-oesophageal reflux.

Table 7.3. Relationship between tests of vagal function

	Lower oesophageal sphincter response to increased intra-abdominal pressure		Gastric secretory response	
	Normal	Abnormal	Normal	Abnormal
Gastric secretory response:				
Normal	9	7	—	—
Abnormal	2	5	—	—
Heart rate variability:				
Normal	9	8	10	6
Abnormal	3	3	5	1

Both tests of gastrointestinal vagal function were abnormal in five of 23 patients, normal in nine, with one impaired in the remainder. There was no significant correlation between the results of these tests in patients with IBS (Table 7.3).

All three tests of vagal function were performed in 22 patients with IBS. The majority of patients (nine) had one abnormal test, in 6, two tests were abnormal. One patient had abnormality in all three tests, while in six subjects all the tests were normal. Cardiac and alimentary vagal function were not closely correlated (Table 7.3).

DISCUSSION

This study has clearly demonstrated that there is an impairment of vagal function in patients with IBS. This could represent a common basis for the association of GOR with IBS. Despite similar resting intragastric and lower oesophageal sphincter pressures, the same increase in intragastric pressure as in controls failed to produce a normal sphincteric response in over half the patients with IBS. Of the nine IBS patients with oesophagitis, four (44%) showed a subnormal response to elevation of intragastric pressure, two (22%) showed impairment of efferent vagal function (as assessed by the gastric secretory study with insulin and pentagastrin) and two (22%) showed subnormal heart variability with deep respiration. These findings are less than the prevalence of abnormal vagal function in patients with reflux oesophagitis; 71% abnormal sphincteric response (Ogilvie *et al.*, 1985), one-quarter to a half with impaired gastric secretory response to insulin/pentagastrin, while a similar number had evidence of cardiac vagal impairment (Heatley *et al.*, 1980; Ogilvie *et al.*, 1985). These differences may reflect the fact that a relatively small number of IBS patients were studied, they were younger and had less severe oesophagitis than those reported by these other workers.

The reason why patients with IBS should have a disorder of vagal function is not evident from this study. No patient had undergone a vagotomy or had evidence of diabetes mellitus. Other conditions associated with a more widespread autonomic impairment were similarly not present; no patient had evidence of postural hypotension, disordered sweating or bladder dysfunction to suggest progressive autonomic failure.

It seems improbable that vagal abnormality is related solely to the presence of GOR since it was present in IBS patients without demonstrable oesophagitis or pathological reflux on 24-hour pH monitoring. This raises the possibility that these autonomic changes may be of importance in the pathogenesis of IBS itself. This is, of course, a matter of some speculation.

We can no longer regard IBS as a motor disorder confined to the large intestine. Abnormalities in small intestinal transit (Cann *et al.*, 1983) and motility (Thompson *et al.*, 1979, Kumar & Wingate, 1985; Kellow & Phillips, 1987), disordered oesophageal motility (Whorwell *et al.*, 1981), pathological GOR (Smart *et al.*, 1986) and abnormal gall bladder function (Braverman, 1987) have all been reported. Such extensive involvement of the gut suggests a common pathogenetic basis—possibly myogenic, or as suggested 60 years ago, neurogenic in origin (Bockus *et al.*, 1928). In the latter, a carefully conducted study involving detailed history, clinical examination and neurological investigation, the authors concluded that 'It is our belief that the aetiology of mucous colitis is in some way linked to the alterations in the function of the vegetative nervous system'.

In this context, it is of interest to compare IBS with conditions associated with abnormal vagal function. Truncal vagotomy was introduced to treat peptic ulceration over 40 years ago and is associated with disordered oesophageal function (Ogilvie & Atkinson, 1984), gastric emptying (Foster *et al.*, 1984) and motility (Malagelada *et al.*, 1980) together with abnormal small bowel (Thompson *et al.*, 1982) and colonic motor function (Connell & McKelvey, 1970), directly due to nerve section. Diabetes mellitus is probably the most common cause of vagal dysfunction encountered in clinical practice, with up to one-third of patients having some autonomic abnormality (Hosking *et al.*, 1978). As with vagotomy, widespread gastrointestinal motor involvement has been described with oesophageal dysfunction (Stewart *et al.*, 1976) impaired gastric emptying (Foster *et al.*, 1984) and motor function (Malagelada *et al.*, 1980) abnormal small intestinal (Camilleri & Malagelada, 1984; Foster *et al.*, 1984) and colonic (Battle *et al.*, 1980) motility.

Structural abnormalities of the autonomic nervous system have been demonstrated in diabetics. This, together with the similarity of the motility changes to those following truncal vagotomy, suggests that the underlying mechanism is one of autonomic nervous dysfunction (Feldman & Schiller, 1983).Whilst cardiac dysfunction is obviously not a recognized consequence of vagotomy, similarities in the patchy denervation seen in diabetics (Hosking *et al.*, 1978) to those apparent in patients with IBS, together with the finding of a similar spectrum of disordered gastrointestinal motility, suggests that vagal impairment may have some role in the genesis of the pathophysiological abnormalities in IBS.

Progressive autonomic failure is becoming increasingly recognized in clinical practice, being manifest as postural hypotension, defective sweating, with impaired bladder and sexual function as a consequence of neuronal cell loss (Bannister, 1983). These primary or secondary syndromes are associated with gastrointestinal dysfunction, with impaired oesophageal (Battle *et al.*, 1979), gastric and small intestinal motility (Camilleri *et al.*, 1985), and colonic (Battle *et al.*, 1979) motor function. These changes, however, differ from those found following vagotomy and in diabetics, in that phase III of the interdigestive migrating motor complex is preserved in those conditions yet lost in progressive autonomic failure. Loss of phase III may represent damage to the enteric nervous system which is responsible for programming this motor phenomenon (Wingate, 1983): no such changes have been described in IBS, in which enteric nervous function appears intact (Kumar & Wingate, 1985).

As well as autonomic impairment, evidence of autonomic arousal also exists in IBS as judged by clinical features (Fielding, 1981) and investigations such as forearm blood flow (Palmer *et al.*, 1974) and cold pressor tests (Fielding & Regan, 1984). One can hypothesize therefore, that this imbalance in the autonomic nervous system, through a combination of efferent and afferent, inhibitory and excitatory changes, could adversely affect the modulation of enteric nervous system programming, producing dysmotility or altered perception of normal gut function, which characterizes the pathophysiological disturbance of IBS.

At the present time this suggestion is purely speculative. This study was designed to investigate vagal function in relation to GOR in IBS and, as such, no motor function outside the oesophagus was assessed. Clearly, changes in autonomic function in IBS must be related to altered patterns of gastrointestinal motility to substantiate this hypothesis. More detailed investigation, perhaps including the study of central and gut nerves, would delineate further the extent and significance of the autonomic abnormality in IBS.

REFERENCES

Atkinson, M., Edwards, D.A.W., Honour, A.J. & Rowlands, E.N. (1957) The oesophago-gastric sphincter in hiatus hernia. *Lancet* ii, 1138–1142.

Bannister, R. (1983) Clinical features of progressive autonomic failure. In Bannister, R. (ed), *Autonomic Failure. A Textbook of Clinical Disorders of the Autonomic Nervous System*, pp. 67–73. Oxford Medical Publications, Oxford.

Battle, W.M., Rubin, M.R., Cohen, S. & Snape, W.J. (1979) Gastrointestinal motility in amyloidosis. *New Engl J Med* 301, 24–25.

Battle, W.M., Snape, W.J., Alavi, A., Cohen, S. & Braunstein, S. (1980) Colonic dysfunction in diabetes mellitus. *Gastroenterology* 79, 1217–1221.

Bennett, T., Farquar, I.R., Hosking, D.J. & Hampton, J.R. (1978) Assessment of methods for estimating autonomic control of the heart in patients with diabetes mellitus. *Diabetes* 27, 1167–1174.

Bockus, H.L., Bank, J. & Wilkinson, S.A. (1928) Neurogenic mucous colitis. *Am J Med Sci* 176, 813–829.

Braverman, D. (1987) Gall bladder contraction in patients with irritable bowel syndrome. *Gut* 28, A1384.

Camilleri, M. & Malagelada, J.R. (1984) Abnormal intestinal motility in diabetics with the gastroparesis syndrome. *Eur J Clin Invest* 14, 420–427.

Camilleri, M., Malagelada, J.R., Stanghellini, V., Fealey, R.D. & Steps, S.G. (1985) Gastrointestinal motility disturbances in patients with orthostatic hypotension. *Gastroenterology* 88, 1852–1859.

Cann, P.A., Read, N.W., Brown, C., Hobson, M. & Holdworth, C.D. (1983) Irritable bowel (colon) syndrome: relationship of disorder in the transit of a single solid meal to symptom patterns. *Gut* 24, 405–411.

Connell, A.M. & McKelvey, S.T.P. (1970) Influence of vagotomy on the colon. *Proc Roy Soc Med* (Suppl) 63, 7–9.

Dodds, W.J., Hogan, W.J., Stef, J.J., Miller, W.N., Lydon, S.B. & Arndorfer, R.C. (1975a) Effect of increased intra-abdominal pressure on lower esophageal sphincter pressure. *Am J Dig Dis* 20, 298–308.

Dodds, W.J., Hogan, W.J., Stef, J.J., Miller, W.N., Lydon, S.B. & Arndorfer, R.C. (1975b) A rapid pull-through technique for measuring lower esophageal sphincter pressure. *Gastroenterology* 68, 437–43.

Dotevall, G., Svedlund, J. & Sjodin, I. (1982) Symptoms in irritable bowel syndrome. *Scand J Gastroenterol* 17 (Suppl 79), 16–19.

Faber, R.G., Russell, R.C.G., Royston, C.M.S., Whitfield, P. & Hobsley, M. (1974) Duodenal reflux during insulin stimulated secretion. *Gut* 15, 880–884.

Feldman M. & Schiller, L.R. (1983) Disorders of gastrointestinal motility associated with diabetes mellitus. *Ann Int Med* 93, 378–384.

Fielding, J.F. (1981) The diagnostic sensitivity of physical signs in irritable bowel syndrome. *Ir Med J* 74, 143–144.

Fielding, J.F. & Regan, R. (1984) Excessive cold pressor responses in the irritable bowel syndrome. *Ir J Med Sci* 153, 356–357.

Foster, G.E., Evans, D.F., Arden-Jones, J.R., Beattie, A. & Hardcastle, J.D. (1984) Abnormal gastrointestinal motility in diabetics and after vagotomy. In Roman, C. (ed), *Gastrointestinal Motility*, pp. 305–310. MTP Press, Lancaster.

Heatley, R.V., Collins, R.J., James, P.D. & Atkinson, M. (1980) Vagal function in relation to gastro-oesophageal reflux and associated motility changes. *Br Med J* 280, 755–757.

Hobsley, M. & Silen, W. (1969) The use of an inert marker (phenol red) to improve accuracy in gastric secretory studies. *Gut* 10, 787–795.

Hosking, D.J., Bennett, T. & Hampton, J.R. (1978) Diabetic autonomic neuropathy. *Diabetes* 27, 1043–1055.

Kellow, J.E. & Phillips, S.F. (1987) Altered small bowel motility in irritable bowel syndrome is correlated with symptoms. *Gastroenterology* 92, 1885–1893.

Kumar, D. & Wingate, D.L. (1985) The irritable bowel syndrome: a paroxysmal motor disorder. *Lancet* ii, 973–977.

MacLaurin, C. (1963) The intrinsic sphincter in the prevention of gastro-oesophageal reflux. *Lancet* ii, 801–805.

Malagelada, J.R., Rees, W.D.W., Mazzotta, L.J. & Go, V.L.W. (1980) Gastric motor abnormalities in diabetic and post-vagotomy gastroparesis; effects of metoclopramide and bethanechol. *Gastroenterology* 78, 286–293.

Manning, A.P., Thompson, W.G., Heaton, K.W. & Morris, A.F. (1978) Towards positive diagnosis of the irritable bowel syndrome. *Br Med J* 2, 653–654.

Nebel, O.T., Fornes, M.C. & Castell, D.O. (1976) Symptomatic gastroesophageal reflux-incidence and precipitating factors. *Dig Dis* 21, 953–956.

Ogilvie, A.L. & Atkinson, M. (1984) Influence of the vagus nerve upon the reflex control of the lower oesophageal sphincter. *Gut* 25, 253–258.

Ogilvie, A.L., James, P.D. & Atkinson, M. (1985) Impairment of vagal function in reflux oesophagitis. *Q J Med* 54, 61–74.

Palmer, R.L., Stonehill, E., Crisp, A.H., Waller, S.L. & Misiewicz, J.J. (1974) Psychological characteristics of patients with the irritable bowel syndrome. *Postgrad Med J* 50, 416–419.

Rubin, L., Wald, A. & Schuster, M.M. (1979) Unrecognized common features of irritable bowel syndrome. *Gastroenterology* 76, 1230(a).

Smart, H.L., Nicholson, D.A. & Atkinson, M. (1986) Gastro-oesophageal reflux in the irritable bowel syndrome. *Gut* 27, 1127–1131.

Stewart, I.M., Hosking, D.J., Preston, B.J. & Atkinson, M. (1976) Oesophageal motor changes in diabetes mellitus. *Thorax* **31**, 278–283.

Thompson, D.G., Laidlaw, J.M. & Wingate, D.L. (1979) Abnormal small bowel motility demonstrated by radiotelemetry in a patient with irritable colon. *Lancet* **ii**, 1321–1323.

Thompson, D.G., Ritchie, H.D. & Wingate D.L. (1982) Patterns of small intestinal motility in duodenal ulcer patients before and after vagotomy. *Gut* **23**, 517–523.

Thompson, W.G. & Heaton, K.W. (1980) Functional bowel disorders in apparently healthy people. *Gastroenterology* **79**, 283–288.

Venables, C.W. (1970) The value of combined pentagastrin insulin test in studies of stomal ulceration. *Br J Surg* **57**, 757–761.

Watson, W.C., Sullivan, S.N., Corke, M. & Rush, D. (1976) Incidence of oesophageal symptoms in patients with irritable bowel syndrome. *Gut* **17**, 827(a).

Watson, W.C., Sullivan, S.N., Corke, M. & Rush, D. (1978) Globus and headache: common symptoms of the irritable bowel syndrome. *Can Med Assoc J* **118**, 387–388.

Wheeler, T. & Watkins, P.J. (1973) Cardiac denervation in diabetes. *Br Med J* **iv**, 584–586.

Whorwell, P.J., Clouter, C. & Smith, C. (1981) Oesophageal manometry in the irritable bowel syndrome. *Br Med J* **1**, 1101–1102.

Whorwell, P.J., McCallum, M., Creed, F.H. & Roberts, C.T. (1986) Non-colonic features of irritable bowel syndrome. *Gut* **27**, 37–40.

Wingate, D.L. (1983) Complex clocks. *Dig Dis Sci* **28**, 1133–1140.

8 The Possible Role of Stress in the Disturbance of Gut Function and Development of Symptoms

D.G. Thompson

INTRODUCTION

The aims of this article are to introduce the reader to recent information concerning the inter-relationships between autonomic arousal, stress and gut function, as they may relate to the development of clinical symptoms.

The contents of the chapter will be restricted to a review of relevant clinical research data which have been conducted in recent years. For earlier information the reader is referred to other reviews on the topic (Thompson, 1988). Other authors in the book will have referred to *in vitro* and animal studies; these are not within the domain of this chapter.

By the end of this chapter it is expected that the reader will realize that a great deal is still to be done to determine the relationships between autonomic stimulation, the development of gut dysfunction and the occurrence of symptoms. Although the area is still largely uncharted, the last 10 years have seen a series of advances which have shed light on the problem and have begun to bring into focus problems for future studies to address.

Relationships between autonomic arousal and gastrointestinal dysfunction

In considering this relationship it is important to be aware of the functional interactions between the factors involved in the disturbance of gastrointestinal function via autonomic arousal. It needs to be appreciated that a number of steps (Fig. 8.1) are interposed between the perception of a stimulus, which is sufficient to arouse the various defensive and adaptive responses which go to make up the 'fight or flight' response (stress), and altered gut function. One of the major responses to the perception of a perturbing stimulus is of course the activation of sympathetic nervous pathways and the synaptic release of noradrenaline, together with secretion of adrenaline from the adrenal glands. While being a major determinant of the physiological response, catecholamines are not the

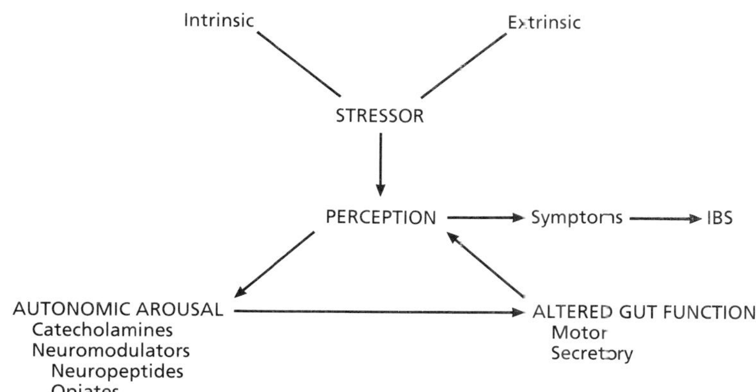

Fig. 8.1. Possible steps between stimulus perception, altered gut function and IBS.

only component, however. It is becoming increasingly recognized that other neurotransmitters and/or modulators are released in response to sympathetic arousal, many of which may influence gut function. Notable among these are neuropeptide Y (Macrae *et al.*, 1986) and somatostatin (Costa & Furness, 1984), both of which are released concomitantly with catecholamines from sympathetic nerves and are capable of profoundly influencing gut function.

The relationship between the release of such neurotransmitters/ neuromodulators and alterations in gut function is now becoming clearer. In most instances the action on gut function appears to be via the intrinsic control mechanisms of the gut rather than the gut itself. Sympathetic nervous fibres synapse with enteric neurones rather than smooth muscles themselves, although smooth muscle cells are provided with β-adrenoreceptors (Hedges & Turner, 1969), stimulation of which (by circulating adrenaline) may induce relaxation.

Relationship between gastrointestinal dysfunction and symptoms

The relationship between autonomically induced alteration in gut function and the development of gut symptoms is the final step of the pathway between stimulus and symptoms and the one which is probably the least well understood. As will be seen from the studies reported below, it is now relatively easy to induce alterations in gut function via experimental autonomic stimulation. The relationship between these measurable alterations in function and the development of symptoms, in either normals or patients presumed to have stress-related disease is, however, by no means clear. Development of strategies to explore this final step remains the great challenge to clinical gastrointestinal physiologists, since it is obvious that it will only be by human study that a true understanding of stress-related gut symptoms can be determined.

HISTORICAL BACKGROUND

Reports of, and association between, autonomic arousal resulting from emotional or other stressful stimulation and changes in gut function go back to the earliest gastroenterological literature. Notable among these are the classical studies of Beaumont (1833), Wolf and Wolff (1944), Almy and Tulin (1947) and Almy, Abbott and Hinkle (1948). Beaumont and Wolf and Wolff each described the function of the stomach of individuals with gastric fistulae, reporting alterations in secretion, motility and mucosal colour under conditions of stress. Almy reported responses of colonic mucosal blood flow and muscular contraction in individuals under more controlled laboratory conditions. In general, all early reports indicated that emotional arousal by whatever means, increased mucosal redness, altered the secretion and influenced the motility of the organs studied. As may be appreciated, however, the restriction of studies to one or two individuals under repeated circumstances, inevitably raises questions about the specificity of the responses. Prospective study of stress, except in certain fortuitous circumstances, was not usually possible and the extent to which an observed event was the result of the alleged stress, or was coincidental, is difficult to determine.

These earlier studies were also conducted without the benefit of current knowledge of normal human intestinal physiology, which is now known to show major differences between fasting and fed activity, together with variation in baseline activity both during the awake and the sleeping state. Unless such predictable cyclical changes are recognized and controlled for, it is obviously difficult for studies to exclude confusion of the data by normal physiological variation.

Recent developments in the study of autonomic arousal and stress

In the last 5–10 years a series of developments, both technical and conceptual, have enabled progress to be made.

Developments in technology

As with the study of cardiac function by the electrocardiogram (ECG), the study of gastrointestinal physiology and in particular gastrointestinal motor physiology has benefited from the development of techniques which allow study under a variety of conditions.

Passive study. Techniques such as intraluminal manometric pressure recording and perfusion techniques are now widely used and have enabled an understanding of resting gut function to be obtained (analogous to the standard 12-lead ECG). Information obtained in the clinical context with these techniques provides information about resting physiology but cannot of course be used to predict abnormalities, e.g. due to sympathetic stimulation, since analysis is usually retrospective.

Dynamic study. These studies (analogous to the exercise ECG) have now brought the understanding of human physiology into areas more relevant for current discussion. A number of experimental stimuli have now been developed which are capable of inducing autonomic stimulation. In many cases these stimuli are also capable of producing measureably altered gastrointestinal function.

Stimuli which have recently been employed include: a version of the cold presser test (O'Brien *et al.*, 1987) (physical stressor); dichotic listening (McRay *et al.*, 1982) (a mental stressor); a number of other 'psychological' stimuli including noise (Erckenbrecht *et al.*, 1985); mental arithmetic tasks and delayed auditory feedback (Valori *et al.*, 1986); and the Stroop colour word discrimination test (Narducci *et al.*, 1985). These techniques attempt prospectively to induce changes in gut function and to uncover abnormalities which might otherwise not be recognized.

Prolonged study. A third technique which has recently been developed is long-term study for periods of 24–48 hours (Kumar & Wingate, 1985). This technique, which is analogous to prolonged (24 hour) ECG monitoring, provides the opportunity to correlate the presence of symptoms with gastrointestinal motor events during unrestricted daily life. Unless there is an attempt to stimulate the gut prospectively, however, it may still be difficult to determine whether the recorded motor abnormality is the cause or the result of the coincident symptoms.

Developments in gut physiology and pharmacology

In addition to these technical innovations, advances in the understanding of gut physiology and pharmacology now provide a more rational basis for the conduct of studies into relationships between stress and gut function. Newer understanding of the adrenoreceptor subtype localization in the gut and the inter-relationship between β-1 and β-2, α-1 and α-2 subtype localizations to different cellular organs (Motulsky & Irsel, 1982; O'Donnell & Wanstall 1987) also now permit more fundamental exploration of stress effects using specific adrenoreceptor agonists and antagonists.

STUDIES ON EXPERIMENTAL STRESS AND HUMAN GUT FUNCTION

The following section reviews some of the recent publications which have attempted to explore the relationship between stress and gut function in both health and disease. This section is not an exhaustive review but is intended to show current areas of research interest and to indicate possible relationships between disturbed physiology and symptom development.

The oesophagus

Symptoms of swallowing difficulty and the sensation of 'something in the throat' are often reported by patients in the absence of recognizable structural abnormality. While some of these patients will possibly, in retrospect, turn out to have subtle, hitherto unrecognized neurological disorders, there is a strong clinical suspicion that in many others a disorder of function is the result of patient distress.

Studies by Cook and colleagues (1986) have attempted to study the response of the upper oesophageal sphincter to experimental stressors, in particular dichotic listening stress. These studies have indicated that upper oesophageal sphincter pressures increase with the application of the stimulus. With duration of the experiment, however, sphincter pressures fell, probably the result of adaptation (always a problem with mental stimuli) in the normal subjects. Further studies, more recently conducted (Soffer *et al.*, 1988), have investigated function in the oesophageal body during a variety of stimuli, without showing evidence of abnormality, although others have found some evidence of increased non-peristaltic activity (Robertson *et al.*, 1988).

It therefore seems that in the normal individual the programming of the oesophageal peristalsis, unlike the rest of the upper gut, is not amenable to external modulation. Studies on patients with oesophageal symptoms with no organic basis have been relatively few, although some insight into possible aetiological mechanisms has recently been provided by Valori *et al.* (1988), who showed that changes in oesophageal motility pattern can be induced experimentally in normal individuals by hyperventilation. Shortly after a period of hyperventilation, oesophageal peristaltic amplitude appears to be significantly increased, and the magnitude of the response is related to degree of alkalosis induced. The changes seen in this study are of interest because they resemble those of the 'nutcracker' oesophagus, an oesophageal manometric pattern characterized by high amplitude peristalsis, which is often observed in patients with functional disorders of the oesophagus and, in particular, non-cardiac chest pain (Benjamin *et al.*, 1982). Since such patients are also known to exhibit neurotic traits, particularly anxiety (Richter *et al.*, 1986), and since anxiety is well known to induce hyperventilation, it may well be that the linking factor is increased neuromuscular sensitivity induced by hyperventilation-related alkalosis.

The stomach

Experimental stress has now been used to study stress effects on both gastric emptying and gastric secretion. Both are measurable by experimental stimuli, in particular hand immersion in cold water (Thompson *et al.*, 1983), which is associated with suppression of gastric function. Studies using mental arithmetic and dichotic listening, however, have generally failed to show similar effects, possibly because the intensity of the stimulus in such cases is somewhat less severe. Interestingly, after the cessation of the stressful cold water stimulus a rebound increase in secretion is evident (Thompson *et al.*, 1983). The exact nature of the mechanism for this rebound increase remains uncertain. It seems unlikely that this delayed effect is purely catecholamine mediated, since catecholamines themselves are inhibitory to secretion (Heylings *et al.*, 1988) and motility (Tarnoky *et al.*, 1986). As stated above, however, it is known that sympathetic activation induces release not only of catecholamines but also of other neurotransmitters and modulators (Tigranian *et al.*, 1980) which may have longer duration of action on the gut and may perhaps be responsible for this more prolonged hypersecretion. It has also been suggested that rebound parasympathetic stimulation may account for the secretion (Barclay & Turnberg 1987).

The pylorus

Recent studies have investigated the effect of experimental stress on pyloric function (Fone *et al.*, 1988). These studies have shown that isolated pyloric contractions in the fasted gut were reliably inhibited. The relationship between this finding and postprandial pyloric function now needs to be determined.

The small intestine

The effects of stress on the small intestine have been studied by both intraluminal pressure activity, using standard manometry techniques, and upper intestinal transit, which provides an intregrated function of motility and secretion. The effect of experimental stimulation of the small intestine by mental stress appears to be inhibition of the normal cyclical fasted pattern (McRay *et al.*, 1982). This disturbance is characterized by the development of greater than normal intervals between successive phase III activity and a corresponding increase in irregular phase II activity.

Similar studies have now been conducted on patients with irritable bowel syndrome (IBS) using prolonged jejunal manometry together with a variety of stimuli (Kumar & Wingate, 1985; Valori *et al.*, 1986). In essence these studies indicate that many patients with IBS show a more florid response to mental stimuli than normal volunteers. The reason for this increased responsiveness, however, remains uncertain. From Fig. 8.1 it may be seen that possible explanations for these changes are many, ranging from an enhanced perception of the stressor to increased responsiveness of the gut to the stimulus. The additional finding that some of these patients also exhibit an aberrant pattern of fasting jejunal motility even when unstimulated by stressors (Kumar & Wingate, 1985) suggests perhaps that the abnormality lies in the gut.

It is more difficult to demonstrate changes in small intestinal motor patterns during the fed state, largely because methods for recognizing alteration in the apparently random pattern of postprandial motility remain relatively crude. Changes in postprandial motor function have however been noted during cold water stimulation (O'Brien *et al.*, 1985; Fone *et al.*, 1988). As might be expected, a general reduction in frequency of contractions occurs. This reduction is not influenced by prior β-blockade, a finding consistent with the concept that sympathetic influences upon patterns of motility are influenced principally by α-receptor mediated pathways acting upon the enteric ganglia.

To avoid difficulties associated with intubation and interpretation of small intestinal motor activity, another approach which has been adopted has been the measurement of orocaecal transit using the non-invasive technique of serial exhaled breath hydrogen sampling (Cann *et al.*, 1983; O'Brien *et al.*, 1987).

Using this technique, disturbances of transit during experimental stress may be demonstrated, the type of response apparently depending upon the test meal employed. For example, the ingestion of a transit marker such as lactulose which passes largely undigested through the gut, is consistently delayed (O'Brien *et al.*, 1987), whereas the transit of more digestable material such as stachyose and raffinose (the consituents of beans and lentils) is accelerated (Cann *et al.*, 1983). These differences may relate to the effects of stress not only upon motility but also upon intraluminal digestion of the nutrient by the intestinal secretions. Inhibition of digestion might result in an overall acceleration of transit if undigested but osmotically active particles are retained within the gut lumen while non-digestible particles (lactulose) would not be similarly affected. Further experiments on transit using a variety of adrenergic agonists and antagonists have now shown that the delaying effect of physical stress on lactulose transit is largely β-adrenoreceptor mediated (O'Brien *et al.*, 1985). This effect can be mimicked by the infusion of isoprenaline, a non-specific β-adrenoreceptor agonist, while prior β-blockade markedly attenuates the cold water effect (McIntyre *et al.*, 1988).

Other recent studies into the role of autonomic sympathetic control of gut function have indicated that, even under non-stimulated conditions, there exists a resting sympathetic influence upon the small intestine which modulates gut transit. It has been shown, for example, that the speed of transit under non-stressful conditions is significantly accelerated by the prior adminstration of β-blockers (McIntyre *et al.*, 1988). The acceleration produced seems moreover to depend upon the pre-existing transit speed, being more rapid with longer intrinsic transit rates.

The colon and rectum

The effects of stress upon the colon and rectum have received less recent study, largely because the definition of normal and abnormal colonic function remains elusive and because suitable techniques for non-invasive measurement of colonic activity are yet to be developed.

Recent studies by Narducci (Narducci *et al.*, 1985) have addressed the problem and shown an increase in myoelectric activity in the distal human colon in response to both cold pain and the Stroop Colour Word test. Although the responses were somewhat inconsistent, similarly inconsistent results have been found by others (Sarna *et al.*, 1982; Schang *et al.*, 1988).

More recent studies of rectosigmoid electrical activity during cold pressor stress (Shabsin *et al.*, 1988) do however indicate that the colon increases its activity, perhaps via sympathetic inhibition of a normally tonic inhibitory pathway. Stool frequency also appears to be increased during experimental stress by a mechanism which seems related to colonic rather than small intestinal disturbances (Erckenbrecht *et al.*, 1985).

Anal sphincter tone also seems to be modulated by stress (Kumar *et al.*, 1988). Both psychological and physical stressors inhibit external sphincter activity but produce a tonic rise in anal canal pressure, reflecting an increase in internal sphincter tone.

CONCLUSIONS

It can be seen from the above review that while a start has been made on the understanding of stress effects and gut function, much still needs to be done. Advance at present is limited by both a lack of suitable techniques for study and a lack of suitable probes capable of investigating the non-catecholamine related responses to stress.

The studies so far performed have also indicated the limitations of passive recording and indicate the value of 'dynamic' studies, although the techniques employed for stimulation are still crude. It must be accepted that the physiologic responses to the experimental stimuli, e.g. mental arithmetic or pain, do not necessarily reproduce the effects of stimuli which induce the stress responses in daily life.

It seems likely that important advances will come from longer-term monitoring and from an ability to reproducibly associate symptoms with an abnormality in gut function.

For further long-term understanding, a number of important more fundamental advances need to be made. At 'basic science' level, a greater understanding of the pharmacological responses to autonomic arousal needs to be achieved so that the role of the non-catecholamine mediated sympathetic responses (e.g. neuropeptide Y and somatostatin mediated responses) can be determined. At the 'clinical science' level, a greater ability to apply controlled reproducible models of autonomic arousal is needed, together with development of better non-invasive techniques for studying the less accessible regions of the gut, particularly the colon. These improvements are particularly necessary since, despite the limitations of human studies, it is evident that only careful experimentation on the human subject will advance our understanding of the relationship between stress, gut disease and clinical symptoms. While animal studies can provide some insight into the broader relationships between stress and gut dysfunction, major species differences in stress response are already emerging which will limit the effectiveness of animal studies as models of the human.

Much also needs to be understood about the pharmacology of the stress response, since observations made on the physiology of the cardiovascular system are not necessarily relevant to gut function. Recently the classification of adrenoreceptors has been challenged on the basis of responses to new adrenoreceptor agonists and antagonists, indicating the presence of previously unreported adrenoreceptor subtypes (Croci *et al.*, 1988). Such advances will undoubtedly pave the way for further clinical developments.

<h2 style="text-align:center">REFERENCES</h2>

Almy, T.P. & Tulin, M. (1947) Alterations in colonic function in man under stress: experimental production of changes simulating the 'irritable colon'. *Gastroenterology* 8, 616–626.

Almy, T.P., Abott, K.E. & Hinkle, L.E. (1950) Alterations in colonic function in man under stress. IV. Hypomotility of the sigmoid colon and its relationship to the mechanism of functional diarrhoea. *Gastroenterology* 15, 95–103.

Barclay, G.R. & Turnberg, L.A. (1987) The effect of psychological stress on salt and water transport in the human jejunum. *Gastroenterology* 93, 91–98.

Beaumont, W. (1833) *Experiments and Observations on the Gastric Juice and the Physiology of Digestion*. F.P. Allen, Plattsburgh.

Benjamin, S.B., Gerhart, D.C. & Castell, D.O. (1982) High-amplitude peristaltic esophageal contractions associated with chest pain and/or dysphagia. *Gastroenterology* 83, 364–370.

Cann, P.A., Read, N.W. & Cammack, J. (1983) Psychological stress and the passage of a standard meal through the stomach and small intestine in man. *Gut* 24, 236–240.

Cook, I.J., Dent, J., Shannon, S., Silletti, C. & Collins, S.M. (1986) Measurement of upper oesophageal sphincter pressure: the effect of stress. *Gastroenterology* 91, A1049.

Costa, M. & Furness, J.B. (1984) Somatostatin is present in a subpopulation of noradrenergic nerve fibres supplying the intestine. *Neuroscine* 13, 911–920.

Croci, T., Giudice, A., Nava, M. *et al.* (1988) Inhibition of colonic motility and cardiovascular effects of new gut-specific β-adrenergic agonists in anaesthetized rats. (Paper presented at the 4th European Symposium on Gastroenterology Motility, Krakow, Poland, 1988).

Erckenbrecht, J.F., Schoepe-Stiller, A., Borges, J., Rehm, S. & Weinbeck, M. (1985) The effect of mental stress by noise on motility and fluid absorption in the human upper small bowel. *Dig Dis Sci* 30, 768.

Fone, D., Horowitz, M., Maddox, A., *et al.* (1988) Cold stress induces isolated pyloric pressure waves in healthy volunteers. *Gastroenterology* 94, A133.

Hedges, A. & Turner, P. (1969) β-Receptors in human isolated smooth muscle. *Br J Pharmacol* 37, 547–548.

Heylings, J.R., Redfern, J.S. & Feldman, M. (1988) Inhibitory effect of isoprenaline on gastric acid secretion in the rat. The role of endogenous histamine. *Aliment Pharm Therap* 2, 419–428.

Kumar, D. & Wingate, D.L. (1985) The irritable bowel syndrome, a paroxysmal motor disorder. *Lancet* ii, 973–977.

Kumar, D., Waldron, D., Williams, N.S. & Wingate, D.L. (1988) The effect of psychological and pain stress on anorectal motility and external sphincter activity in humans. *Hepatogastroenterology* 35, 182.

Macrae, I.M., Furness, J.B. & Costa, M. (1986) Distribution of subgroups of noradrenaline neurones in the coeliac ganglion of the guinea pig. *Cell Tissue Res* 244, 173–180.

McIntyre, A.S., Thompson, D.G., Burnham, W.R. & Walker, E. (1988) The mode of action and functional consequence of β-adrenergic tone in the human gut. *Gastroenterology* 94, A296.

McRay, S., Younger, K., Thompson, D.G. & Wingate, D.L. (1982) Sustained mental stress alters human jejunal motor activity. *Gut* 23, 404–409.

Motulsky, J.H. & Irsel, P.A. (1982) Adrenergic receptors in man. *New Engl J Med* 307, 18–29.

Narducci, F., Snape, W.J., Battle, W.M., London, R.L. & Cohen, S. (1985) Increased colonic motility during exposure to a stressful situation. *Dig Dis Sci* 30, 40–44.

O'Brien, J.D., Thompson, D.G., Holly, J., Burnham, W.R. & Walker, E. (1985) Stress disturbs human gastrointestinal transit via a β1-adrenoreceptor mediated pathway. *Gastroenterology* 88, A1520.

O'Brien, J.D., Thompson, D.G., Burnham, W.R., Holly, J. & Walker, E. (1987) Action of centrally mediated autonomic stimulation on human gastrointestinal transit: a comparative study of two stimuli. *Gut* 28, 960–969.

O'Donnell, S.R. & Wanstall, J.C. (1987) Functional evidence for differential regulation of β-adrenoreceptor subtypes. *TIPS* 8, 265–268.

Richter, J.E., Obrecht, F., Bradley, L.A., Young, L.D. & Anderson, K.O. (1986) Psychological comparison of patients with nutcracker esophagus or irritable bowel syndrome. *Dig Dis Sci* 31, 131–138.

Robertson, D.A., Naylor, K., Ayres, R. & Smith, C.L. (1988) Acute stress affects oesophageal function. *Gut* 29, A1491–1492.

Sarna, S., Latimer, P., Campbell, D. & Waterfall, W.E. (1982) Effect of stress, meal and neostigmine on rectosigmoid electrical control activity in normals and in irritable bowel syndrome patients. *Dig Dis Sci* 27, 582–591.

Schang, J-C., Devroede, G., Hebert, M., Hemond, H., Pilote, M. & Devroede, L. (1988) Effects of rest, stress and food on myoelectric spiking activity of left and sigmoid colon in humans. *Dig Dis Sci* 33, 614–618.

Shabsin, H., Whitehead, W.E., Enck, P. & Schuster, M. (1988) A comparison of colonic spikes between IBS patients and normals during colon distension, cold pressor stress, and postprandial period. *Gastroenterology* **94**, A421.

Soffer, E.E., Scalabrini, P., Pope, C.E. & Wingate, D.L. (1988) Effects of stress on oesophageal motor function in normal subjects and in patients with irritable bowel syndrome. *Gut* **29**, 1591–1594.

Tarnoky, K., Szenohradszky, J. & Petri, G. (1986) Changes in small bowel motility and noradrenaline content of the intestinal wall in response to α- and β-adrenergic blockade in dog. *Acta Physiol Hung* **67**, 447–456.

Thompson, D.G., Richelson, E. & Malagelada, J.R. (1983) Perturbation of upper gastrointestinal function by cold stress. *Gut* **24**, 277–283.

Thompson, D.G. (1988) Central control of human gastrointestinal function. In Read, N.J. & Grundy, D. (eds), *Baillière's Clinical Gastroenterology 2*, pp. 107–123. Baillière Tindall, London.

Tigranian, R.A., Orloff, L., Kalita, N.F., Davydova, N.A. & Pavlova, E.A. (1980) Changes in blood levels of several hormones, catecholamines, prostaglandins, electrolytes and cAMP in man during emotional stress. *Endocrinol Exp* **14**, 101–112.

Valori, R.M., Kumar, D. & Wingate, D.L. (1986) Effects of different types of stress and of 'prokinetic' drugs on the control of the fasting motor complex in humans. *Gastroenterology* **90**, 1890–1900.

Valori, R.M., Cole, E., Lemon, M., Howard, R. & Cockel, R. (1988) Hyperventilation increases the amplitude of oesophageal contractions in healthy volunteers: a controlled study. *Gut* **29**, A1447.

Wolf, S. & Wolff, H.G. (1944) *Human Gastric Function, an Experimental Study of a Man and his Stomach*. Oxford University Press, New York.

9 *Gut Sensitivity*

F. Cervero

INTRODUCTION

Abdominal pain is a symptom frequently reported by patients suffering from irritable bowel syndrome (IBS). However, numerous anatomical and functional investigations in these patients have failed to find a unique gut lesion to which the feeling of pain could be attributed. It is conceivable that the abdominal pain felt by IBS patients could be the consequence of an increased sensory awareness induced by a more excitable central nervous system (CNS). If this is the case, then the symptom of abdominal pain would not be due to a peripheral lesion but to an abnormal CNS, and it is well known that some neurological and psychological disorders induce such central alterations of pain perception. However, it is also possible that functional disorders at the bowel level, including motor and biochemical dysfunctions, could result in the activation of sensory receptors in the gut responsible for the triggering of pain sensations. For instance, increased or abnormal motility can evoke colicky pain, as can the presence within the environment of the sensory receptors of compounds such as histamine, serotonin or certain neuropeptides. For the purposes of this chapter I will deal exclusively with those forms of peripheral activation of the sensory pathways that mediate the feeling of abdominal pain, particularly of gut pain. However, one must bear in mind that there may be an important central component in the abdominal pain felt by IBS patients, and that this central component could be part of a more general dysfunction of the CNS to which symptoms other than pain can also be attributed. (For a more detailed account of the peripheral and central mechanisms of gastrointestinal pain, see Cervero, 1988.)

In this chapter I will review some aspects of the sensory innervation of the gut, particularly in relation to the perception of pain. The functional properties of sensory receptors in the gut, their mechanisms of activation and the effects of alterations in their environment will be considered. The experimental information available on the functional properties of visceral sensory receptors has sometimes been obtained from viscera belonging to other internal systems (such as the genitourinary system). Therefore, and when appropriate, analogies will be drawn between the innervation of the gut and that of other viscera.

SENSORY INNERVATION OF THE GUT

Sensory receptors in the walls of the gut or in the mesenteries are connected to two different kinds of afferent nerve fibre. Some of these afferent fibres have their nerve cell bodies in the gut, within the submucosal and myenteric plexi of the enteric nervous system (ENS). It is generally thought that these neurones of the ENS do not send axonal projections to the CNS. The area of influence of this kind of afferent neurone is limited to the enteric plexus or includes, at most, the prevertebral ganglia of the autonomic nervous system (ANS) where their axonal projections make contact with postganglionic efferent neurones (Szurszewski, 1981). For this reason it is unlikely that myenteric afferent neurones could play a direct role in the transmission of sensory nociceptive information to the CNS.

The second group of gut afferent neurones have their cell bodies in spinal and cranial ganglia. Their peripheral branches run in sympathetic and parasympathetic nerves and their central projections reach the brainstem and the spinal cord. These afferent neurones are part of a primary afferent system similar to that innervating the skin and other somatic structures. Clinical studies using a combination of stimulation and blocking techniques have repeatedly shown that abdominal pain is evoked by stimulation of sympathetic but not of parasympathetic nerves, and is relieved by section or blockade of sympathetic but not of parasympathetic nerve trunks (White, 1943). Therefore, it seems that most forms of gastrointestinal pain are signalled by afferent fibres in sympathetic nerves, and that the afferent innervation mediated by parasympathetic nerves is principally concerned with regulatory, but not sensory, aspects of gut physiology.

PERIPHERAL INFLUENCES ON GUT SENSORY RECEPTORS

Most of the functional alterations of the gut observed in patients suffering from IBS are probably the consequence of abnormal reflex activity. It is often the case that altered patterns of gut motility and secretion are interpreted as failures of the effector mechanism, i.e. the smooth muscle cell, the secretory cell or the efferent innervation of these two elements. Yet it is not always considered that an abnormal efferent activity can be triggered by afferent signals generated by the activation of sensory receptors which are either

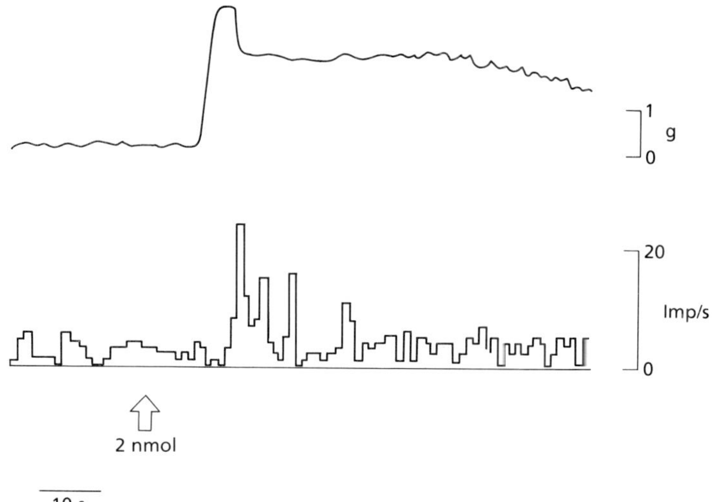

Fig. 9.1. The response of an afferent fibre from the rat's small intestine to intra-arterial injection of substance P (2 nmol). Note that afferent activity was preceded by an increase in tension. Imp/s = impulses per second. (Redrawn with permission from Cervero & Sharkey, 1988.)

sensitized or desensitized. It is, indeed, possible to evoke an abnormal reflex mediated by a perfectly normal smooth muscle or secretory cell, but one that is responding to an abnormal afferent barrage. This interpretation can also help to explain the sensory symptom of IBS, i.e. the abdominal pain, as a consequence of altered responsiveness of the sensory receptor.

These two different mechanisms of activation of a local motor reflex in the gut have been demonstrated in a recent experimental study of the sensory innervation of the small intestine of the rat (Cervero & Sharkey, 1988). Using an *in vitro* preparation of rat ileum with an intact nerve supply, it was possible to observe the responses of sensory receptors in the gut to mechanical stimulation of the intestine and to the application of biologically active compounds (Figs 9.1 & 9.2). For instance, intra-arterial injection of substance P resulted in an excitation of the afferent fibre that appeared as a consequence of the smooth muscle contraction induced by substance P (Fig. 9.1). In this case it is clear that substance P, normally released from intestinal afferent fibres following intense stimulation, had a direct action on the smooth muscle of the intestine, and that the response of the sensory receptor followed the contraction of the gut. This is therefore an indirect action on the afferent fibre induced by an effector mechanism.

However, in other cases, such as with the application of bradykinin, the response of the receptor preceded the contraction of the muscle (Fig. 9.2). This indicates a direct mechanism of action of this compound on the sensory terminals, which in turn trigger a local

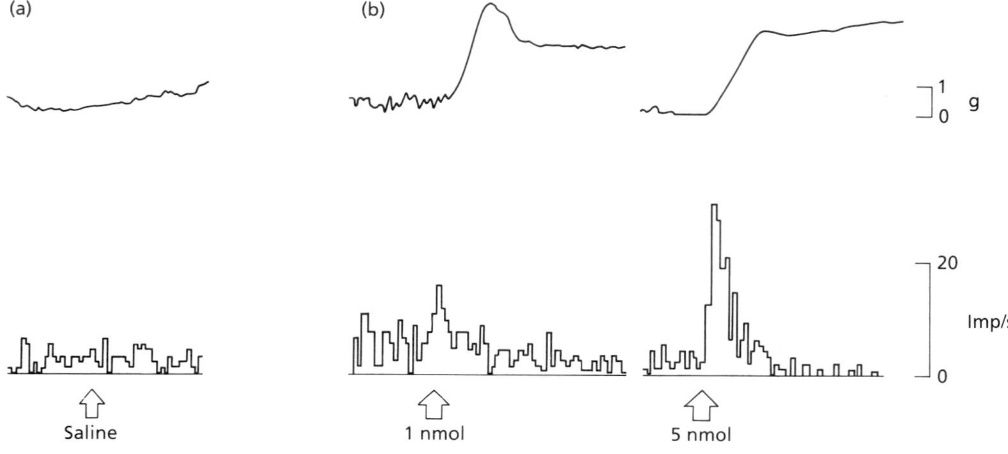

Fig. 9.2. The responses of an afferent fibre from the rat's small intestine to intra-arterial injection of (a) a saline control, and (b) bradykinin at the doses shown. Note that tension in the smooth muscle increases always after the increase in activity of the afferent fibre. Imp/s = impulses per second. (Redrawn with permission from Cervero & Sharkey, 1988.)

reflex observed as a contraction of the smooth muscle. In this case the origin of the effect is in the sensory receptor and the activation of the muscle is a consequence of the discharge induced by bradykinin in the sensory receptor.

These results show that functional alterations of gut motility and secretion can be the consequence of either an abnormal functioning of the effector cells, or of changes in the responsiveness of the sensory receptors in the gut which are normally responsible for the triggering of local reflex action. Both forms of alteration can coexist and both can be induced by the release of naturally occurring compounds in the gut, such as bradykinin or substance P.

SENSITIZATION OF VISCERAL NOCICEPTORS

There are essentially two different mechanisms for the encoding of visceral nociceptive events.

1 Receptors responsible for the sensations of visceral pain are the same population of visceral receptors responding to innocuous stimuli and responsible for visceral reflex actions. These receptors respond to noxious stimuli with higher frequencies of firing.

2 Receptors responsible for the sensations of visceral pain are a different population of visceral receptors which respond to the same stimuli that evoke visceral reflex actions but with different thresholds or by different mechanisms. This view postulates the existence of specific visceral nociceptors.

There is experimental evidence for the existence in the gut of both specific nociceptors and non-specific sensory receptors (see Jänig & Morrison, 1986). High threshold receptors have been described in the biliary system responding to intense mechanical stimulation of the gall bladder and bile ducts (Cervero, 1982). The colon appears to be innervated by small myelinated afferent fibres with a wide range of mechanical thresholds (Blumberg *et al.*, 1983) and by unmyelinated afferent fibres with high mechanical thresholds. In addition, many gut afferents are chemosensitive and can be easily activated by compounds such as bradykinin or histamine, which are naturally released by local tissue damage or inflammation.

One possible mechanism for the feeling of abdominal pain and the functional disorders of gut motility associated with IBS could be the sensitization of gut nociceptors. According to this inter-pretation, gut nociceptors—which normally have a relatively high threshold and respond only to intense forms of stimulation—become abnormally sensitive by decreasing their threshold for activation, thus being sensitive to mild forms of stimulation. As a result, gut reflex activity, normally triggered only by a strong stimulus, appears now as a result of the ordinary physiological process of digestion. This disrupts digestive patterns, evokes ab-normal gut motility and secretion and leads to the perception of abdominal pain.

This interpretation fits well with the concept of a gut that has become abnormal by giving exaggerated responses to mild stimuli. The intestinal responses are appropriate and always due to the activation of functionally adequate reflex pathways. However, as the sensory receptors are sensitized, such responses are exaggerated and out of proportion in relation to the originating stimulus.

There is considerable experimental evidence in support of the idea of sensitization of visceral nociceptors. For instance, Haupt *et al.* (1983) have shown that sensory receptors in the colon of the cat become spontaneously active as a consequence of ischaemia of the gut. In this study, ischaemia of the colon induced an increased and irregular spontaneous activity in the sensory receptors, which became also sensitized to pressure and chemical stimuli.

In a study of the afferent innervation of the ureter, Cervero and Sann (1989) have also demonstrated a similar mechanism. They used an *in vitro* preparation of the guinea-pig ureter with an intact nerve supply, and measured the distension thresholds of mechano-sensitive afferent fibres with receptive fields in the wall of the ureter. They found that, if the ureter was not perfused intraluminally with oxygenated fluid, the spontaneous activity of the afferent fibres was higher and their pressure thresholds were lower than in prepara-tions in which the ureters were perfused with oxygenated fluid at a physiological flow rate (Fig. 9.3). They concluded that an

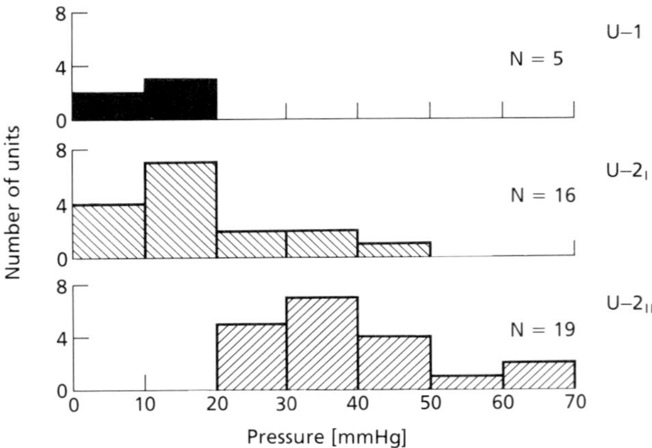

Fig. 9.3. Distributions of the response thresholds to intraluminal pressure increases of ureteric afferent fibres. Top: U-1 fibres with low thresholds; Middle: U-2$_I$ fibres recorded in preparations without intraluminal perfusion; Bottom: U-2$_{II}$ fibres recorded in preparations with intraluminal perfusion. (Redrawn with permission from Cervero & Sann, 1989.)

insufficient oxygen supply, reproducing the conditions of *in vivo* ischaemia, sensitized the high threshold nociceptors in the ureter to a lower threshold and to a greater responsiveness. This study, in a viscus outside the gastrointestinal tract, shows that sensitization of visceral nociceptors is a widespread feature of the innervation of several internal organs and can be responsible for exaggerated responses of the viscera to normal forms of stimulation.

SILENT NOCICEPTORS

Over the last few years, a number of experimental studies on the innervation of deep and visceral structures have provided evidence for the existence of sensory receptors that are only activated by persistent damage or inflammation of the tissue that they innervate. These are believed to be silent nociceptors, normally unresponsive to physiological forms of stimulation and only coming into activation when the tissue suffers persistent damage.

If such silent nociceptors were to be brought into action in patients suffering from IBS, this could explain the symptoms of abdominal pain and the abnormal reflex activity of the gut. This interpretation is in line with the concept of a new or normally not present mechanism being responsible for the abnormal gut. When silent nociceptors are activated, new reflexes develop and the CNS receives information not previously available. Therefore, these are not exaggerated responses to a normal stimulus but entirely new responses induced by novel sensory signals.

The best evidence so far for the existence of silent nociceptors comes from studies on the sensory innervation of the joints. The properties of articular sensory receptors have been examined using a model of experimental arthritis in which the knee joint of the cat undergoes acute inflammation following the injection of kaolin and carrageenin (Schaible & Schmidt, 1985). Using this model, Schaible and Schmidt (1988) have described the existence of unmyelinated afferent fibres in the knee joint which are unresponsive to innocuous and noxious stimulation of the joint in the normal state, but that become sensitive to such movements within a few hours of the induction of experimental arthritis. Their evidence shows that these receptors were quite insensitive prior to the inflammation and highly responsive to normal articular movements once the inflammation developed.

This kind of silent nociceptor has also been found in the colon and urinary bladder (W. Jänig, personal communication). In these studies, still in progress, receptors in the wall of the bladder were found which could not be activated in the normal state but that became responsive to bladder distension and contraction following the induction of an inflammation of the bladder with turpentine.

Although there is still no direct evidence for such a silent nociceptor in the small intestine, the fact that these receptors have been found in different organs and in several locations would suggest that they may represent a general category of sensory receptor. However, their possible role in gut sensory and motor mechanisms and in the physiopathology of conditions such as IBS remains, at present, speculative.

CONCLUSIONS

There is no doubt that a number of gut alterations can result in the perception of abdominal pain and that some of these dysfunctions could account for the pain reported by IBS patients. However, since the pathophysiology of IBS is not yet fully understood, and neurological and psychological syndromes can also result in abnormal pain perception, it is necessary to keep in mind that the abdominal pain felt by IBS patients could have an important central component. The extent and relevance of peripheral vs. central factors in the genesis of IBS pain remains to be established.

Functional alterations of gut motility and secretion can be due to dysfunction of the effector cell and/or to abnormal sensitivity of sensory receptors. The latter can be the consequence of a direct action of peripherally released compounds on the sensory endings. Such abnormal sensitivity can then evoke reflex actions in the gut that are either inappropriate or exaggerated.

There is considerable experimental evidence in favour of the concept of sensitization of visceral nociceptors. This implies a reduction in the activation threshold of visceral nociceptors and an increase in their excitability. Sensitized nociceptors are thus able to respond to innocuous stimuli which may then evoke pain and abnormal reflex actions.

Recent studies using experimental models of inflammation have demonstrated the existence of silent nociceptors, i.e. nociceptors that are normally unresponsive but that come into play as a result of prolonged stimulation or inflammation. Such category of sensory receptor could be responsible for some of the symptoms of IBS by evoking an abnormal reflex and sensory activity as a consequence of a persistent peripheral lesion (functional or anatomical) of the gut.

REFERENCES

Blumberg, H., Haupt, P., Jänig, W. & Kohler, W. (1983) Encoding of visceral noxious stimuli in the discharge patterns of visceral afferent fibres from the colon. *Pflügers Archiv* **398**, 33–40.

Cervero, F. (1982) Afferent activity evoked by natural stimulation of the biliary system in the ferret. *Pain* **13**, 137–151.

Cervero, F. (1988) Neurophysiology of gastrointestinal pain. In Read, N.J. & Grundy, D. (eds), *Ballière's Clinical Gastroenterology 2, Neurophysiology of the Gut*, pp. 183–199. Baillière Tindall, London.

Cervero, F. & Sann, H. (1989) Mechanically evoked responses of afferent fibres innervating the guinea-pig's ureter: an *in vitro* study. *J Physiol* **412**, 245–266.

Cervero, F. & Sharkey, K.A. (1988) An electrophysiological and anatomical study of intestinal afferent fibres in the rat. *J Physiol* **401**, 381–397.

Haupt, P., Jänig, W. & Kohler, W. (1983) Response pattern of visceral afferent fibres supplying the colon upon chemical and mechanical stimuli. *Pflügers Archiv* **398**, 41–47.

Jänig, W. & Morrison, J.F.B. (1986) Functional properties of spinal visceral afferents supplying abdominal and pelvic organs with special emphasis on visceral nociceptors. In Cervero, F. & Morrison, J.F.B. (eds), *Visceral Sensation, Progress in Brain Research* Vol. 67, pp. 87–114. Elsevier, Amsterdam.

Schaible, H.G. & Schmidt, R.F. (1985) Effects of an experimental arthritis on the sensory properties of fine articular afferent units. *J Neurophysiol* **54**, 1109–1122.

Schaible, H.G. & Schmidt, R.F. (1988) Direct observation of the sensitization of articular afferents during an experimental arthritis. In Dubner, R. *et al.* (eds), *Proceedings of the Vth World Congress on Pain*, pp. 44–50. Elsevier, Amsterdam.

Szurszewski, J.H. (1981) Physiology of mammalian prevertebral ganglia. *Ann Rev Physiol* **43**, 53–68.

White, J.C. (1943) Sensory innervation of the viscera. *Res Publ Ass Res Nerv Men Dis* **23**, 273–390.

10 *Modulation of Visceral Afferent Activity as a Therapeutic Possibility for Gastrointestinal Disorders*

P.L.R. Andrews

INTRODUCTION

Therapies for gastrointestinal disorders, whether they be of motility or secretion, have tended to follow three main lines.

1 Antagonism of identified receptors usually involved in producing a stimulation of the activity in a target tissue; examples of this approach include antagonism of histamine-H_2 receptors on gastric oxyntic cells by cimetidine or ranitidine, and muscarinic cholinergic receptors on smooth muscle cells by atropine and its derivatives.

2 Compounds have been developed which are either receptor agonists on the smooth muscle cells (e.g. carbachol), or which evoke the release of neurotransmitter from the enteric nervous system (ENS), for example the substituted benzamides (e.g. metoclopramide, cisapride, Renzapride), which are thought to facilitate the release of acetylcholine from the ENS, stimulating gastrointestinal motility and hence gastric emptying. Prostaglandin analogues used to enhance cytoprotection in the gut may also be considered to be examples of this type of approach.

3 The most recent approach has been to design drugs to directly influence the permeability of the smooth muscle cell membrane to calcium (e.g. verapamil or related agents), facilitating relaxation of segments of gut in spasm. These agents, which are used to relax vascular smooth muscle, have had a degree of success in the gut (e.g. in 'nutcracker' oesophagus). Another example of this 'cellular' approach are the proton pump blockers such as omeprazol, which have pronounced effects on gastric acid secretion.

Each of these pharmacological approaches has its merits but there are striking differences in the degree of success achieved in different clinical situations. Two particularly contrasting areas are the differences in the success of pharmacological therapy for gastric secretory and motility disorders. Whilst disorders involving the excess secretion of gastric acid can be readily and effectively treated by therapies with a well characterized physiological and pharmacological basis, those in which motility is disordered are far less successfully treated. Even now we do not fully understand the mechanism of action of some gastrokinetic agents which have been in use for many years (e.g. domperidone, metoclopromide—for a discussion of the mechanisms of prokinetic agents, see review by Sanger and King, 1988). One reason why motility disorders may respond so poorly to current therapies is that the pathophysiological and pharmacological bases of many motor disorders are not very well understood and hence it is difficult to know whether agonist- or antagonist-based therapy should be used and at which receptor types it should be targeted. In addition there is an overwhelming assumption, particularly in the clinical literature, that a decrease in motility is due to a defect in the cholinergic system and hence should be treated using a cholinomimetic. Decreased motility could equally be due to increased activity in the non-adrenergic non-cholinergic inhibitory system (Andrews, 1986a).

The treatment of gut motor disturbances represents a major clinical problem, not only because of the changes in gut function they may produce (e.g. reflux, constipation) but also because of the aberrant visceral sensations they may give rise to (e.g. early satiety), which in turn may facilitate the development of ingestive disorders (e.g. anorexia nervosa). One therapeutic approach to gut motor and other disturbances that has received little serious attention is the pharmacological modulation of abdominal visceral afferent activity. This chapter will discuss the possibility of modifying visceral afferent signals to correct abnormal visceral sensations or reflexly evoked abnormal motility patterns. Additionally, the possibility of activation or sensitization of afferents as a therapeutic approach to some gut disorders is reviewed. At present few direct studies to investigate these possibilities have been undertaken and therefore much of this chapter is speculative, although some of the principles involved can be illustrated from the recent studies of the antiemetic properties of 5-hydroxytryptamine ($5HT_3$) receptor antagonists (e.g. Bermudez *et al.*, 1988).

WHY ATTEMPT TO MODIFY VISCERAL AFFERENT ACTIVITY?

The simple answer to this question is that as we do not have totally effective therapies for many gut disorders using conventional approaches, any novel approach is worthy of consideration. However, apart from this there are several sounder reasons why afferent manipulation may be a fruitful approach to some gut problems. One of the major reasons derives from a consideration of the functions of the afferents. Activation of a single set of afferents in one gut region may have widespread effects on several organ systems (see below). If afferent traffic becomes abnormal (see p. 105 for mechanisms) then it is easy to see how this may give rise to

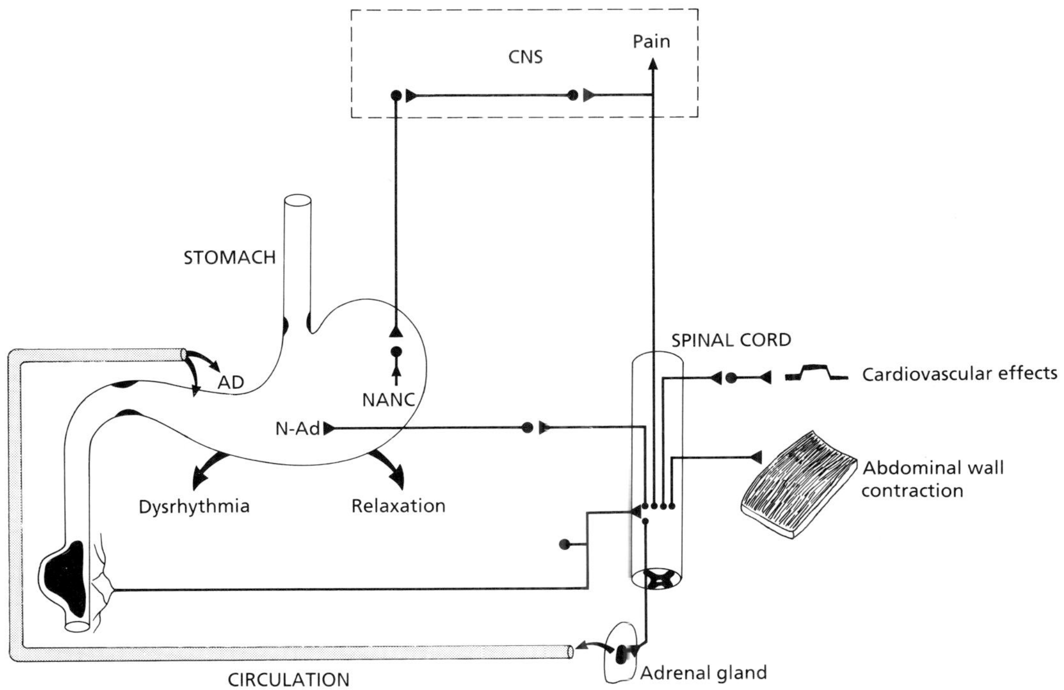

Fig. 10.1. A summary of some of the visceral, somatic and sensory consequences of distension of the intestine, as might be caused by intestinal obstruction. Each effect could be antagonized by a different drug, but all effects could be prevented by blockade of the afferent activated by the distensive stimulus. AD = adrenaline; CNS = central nervous system; N-Ad = noradrenaline from a splanchnic efferent nerve; NANC = non-adrenergic non-cholinergic inhibiting nerve activated by vagal efferents.

the confusing clinical picture manifest in many organ systems, including the CNS. The conventional therapeutic approach is to treat each symptom, often leading to treatment with a 'cocktail' of drugs, but a more rational therapy would be to restore the afferent to normal, thus treating all the symptoms in a single action. This approach is illustrated in Fig. 10.1, which considers the rather extreme example of gut obstruction. Another reason for manipulating afferents is in conditions in which the afferents are hypo- rather than hyperactive. In such conditions pharmacological agents that activate or sensitize afferents could be used to reflexly activate extrinsic vagal efferents supplying, for example, gastric muscle to alleviate gastric stasis. The advantage that this has over conventional approaches is that, because the efferents are being activated reflexly (over the central pathways involved in the genesis of normal efferent patterns), the resulting motility should be identical to that resulting from natural activation of that set of afferents. Similar arguments can be made for reflexes mediated by the ENS or indeed for drugs acting on medullary or hypothalamic neurones which influence the autonomic motor outflows to the gut (e.g. baclofen; Andrews and Wood, 1986).

The above justification for giving serious consideration to drugs influencing afferent activity relies on the presence of gut disorders in which disordered afferent function is a major contributing factor. What is known of the factors influencing the sensitivity of afferents so that predictions can be made about possible afferent involvement in various gut disorders, and is there any clinical evidence for a substantial involvement of afferents in the aetiology of any gastro-intestinal disease? Before discussing these questions it is necessary to outline the functions, anatomical features and properties of the visceral afferent innervation. Where possible we have attempted to illustrate these various aspects using clinical examples from the stomach and colon.

FUNCTIONS OF EXTRINSIC AND INTRINSIC AFFERENTS

Extrinsic afferents

The major functions in which abdominal visceral afferents participate are outlined below, and the organization of the main types of reflex is illustrated in Fig. 10.2.

Viscerovisceral reflexes

This type of reflex is the major one involved in the regulation of gastrointestinal function and may have both the afferent and efferent limbs in the vagus or splanchnic nerves, or the afferent may be in one nerve and the efferent in the other. An example of a vagovagal reflex is the corpoantral reflex (Andrews *et al.*, 1980) in which distension of the gastric body evokes a reflex stimulation of antral contractile activity via the vagus. Distension of the gastric body evokes a reflex relaxation of the gastric body via a vagovagal reflex involving vagal efferent activation of the intramural non-adrenergic non-cholinergic intramural inhibitory neurones (see Andrews, 1986a for review of this reflex). This reflex is involved in the storage of food in the stomach following a meal. In addition to reflexes involving a single gut region, extrinsic reflexes also serve to coordinate activity between gut regions and allow interorgan communication. An example of this type of reflex is a component of the inhibition of gastric motility produced by duodenal distension via a splanchnosplanchnic reflex and probably involved in the duodenal regulation of gastric emptying (Andrews & Lawes, 1984).

Components of the gastrocolic and gastropancreatic reflexes represent other examples of this neurally mediated interorgan

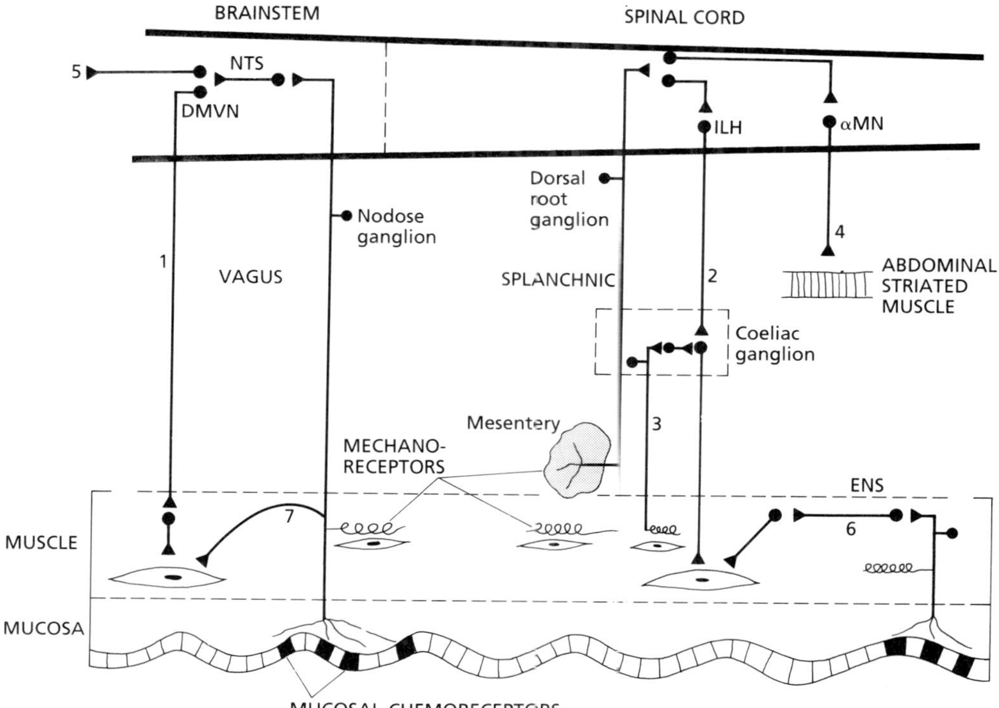

Fig. 10.2. Diagrammatic summary of some of the reflexes controlling gut motility. (1) Vagal efferent activated by a vagal afferent. (2) Splanchnic efferent activated by a splanchnic afferent. (3) Prevertebral reflex, activation of postganglionic sympathetic efferent by a splanchnic afferent via the coeliac ganglion. (4) Activation of somatic efferent α-motor neurone (αMN) by a splanchnic afferent; this is an example of a viscerosomatic reflex. (5) Central projection of vagal afferent information giving rise to some visceral sensations. (6) Intramural reflex mediated by the ENS. (7) Axon collateral of a vagal afferent giving rise to an axon reflex. Note that although muscle mechano- and mucosal chemoreceptors are shown as extensions of the same axon, in practice this information is conveyed in separate axons. DMVN = dorsal motor nucleus of the vagus; ENS = enteric nervous system; NTS = nucleus tractus solitarius; ILH = intermediate lateral horn of the spinal cord.

communication (Harper *et al.*, 1959; Wiley *et al.*, 1988). As well as reflexes linking different gut regions, reflexes are also present which link other systems with the gut. For example, cardiac afferent stimulation evokes reflex relaxation of the gastric body (Abrahamsson & Thoren, 1973) and cardiovascular afferents are presumably involved in the sympathetic modification of gut blood flow during exercise. Activation of gut afferents has widespread effects on other organ systems and such effects may help to explain some of the extragastrointestinal symptoms of gut disorders. Gastric irritation by chemicals can reflexly stimulate airway secretion and increase heart rate, blood pressure vascular resistance and myocardial contractility in the cat (Longhurst *et al.*, 1980, 1981;

German *et al.*, 1982). Gastric distension alone can produce changes in cardiovascular function in the rat and cat (Grundy & Davison, 1981; Longhurst *et al.*, 1981). Could such reflexes be involved in respiratory arrest associated with gastro-oesophageal reflux and sudden death syndrome in infants (Leape *et al.*, 1977) or in postprandial angina? In addition to reflexes influencing the smooth muscle and exocrine tissue of the gut, visceral afferents are also involved in the control of gut and other endocrine secretions. Stimulation of splanchnic afferents evokes a reflex sympathetic discharge to the adrenal medulla. Stimulation of the splanchnic nerves to the adrenal gland evokes the release of adrenaline and enkephalin-like peptides (Govoni *et al.*, 1981) and, as with vaso-pressin (see below), these could have direct effects on gut motility, secretion or absorption via the circulation. In addition to these effects, catecholamines can influence the release of 5HT from the gut enterochromaffin cells and may further influence gut function by this mechanism (Gronstad *et al.* 1988).

One additional type of reflex that requires consideration here is the axon reflex. In this type of reflex some extrinsic afferent axons have an axon collateral, which synapses in the gut wall to influence secretion of bicarbonate ions in the stomach, gastric motility or blood flow, probably via the release of substance P (Fandriks & Delbro, 1983; Delbro *et al.*, 1983, 1984). Further studies are required to assess the significance of this type of reflex in the control of gut function. By analogy with the involvement of axon reflexes in the flare and wheal responses in the skin, where local vasodilatation and increased vascular permeability occur, axon reflexes in the gut may have an important role to play in the local response to mucosal damage. One particularly interesting feature of the abdominal vagal afferents concerns their axonal transport of peptides. Substance P, cholecyclokinin (CCK-8) and somatostatin are synthesized in the cell bodies of the bipolar vagal afferent axons located in the nodose ganglion, with the vast majority of the material (80%?) being transported in the axons towards the gut rather than the medulla (Dockray & Sharkey, 1986). One function of these peripherally transported peptides is to act as neurotrans-mitters and/or neuromodulators in axon reflexes, but could an additional reason for such a large periperal transport be that these peptides have a trophic effect on the gut tissue?

At this point it is worth remembering that, whilst this review is concerned mainly with the possible involvement of visceral afferents in the pathophysiology of gut motility disorders, it is the visceral efferents which generate the abnormal motor patterns in the target tissue in response to the aberrant afferent signal. If this idea is extended, it can be seen that any gut function that is under extrinsic (or intrinsic) efferent influence is potentially accessible to mani-pulation by modification of afferent influences.

In addition to reflexes with the efferent limb in the autonomic nervous system, abdominal visceral afferents can also activate somatic efferents.

The most important example of such a reflex is the abdominal vagal afferent activation of the emetic reflex, involving the rhythmic contraction of the diaphragm and abdominal muscles to compress the stomach and so eject the gastric contents through the mouth. These afferents are involved in the activation of vomiting by ingested agents, e.g. 1 mol/litre NaCl (Andrews & Wood, 1988), whole body radiation (Andrews & Hawthorn, 1987, 1988) and cancer chemotherapeutic agents (Andrews *et al.*, 1988; Hawthorn *et al.*, 1988b). An example of a viscerosomatic reflex involving splanchnic afferents is the 'guarding reaction', in which splanchnic afferent activation produces tensing or contraction of the abdominal muscle overlaying the area from which the afferents originated.

Visceral afferent influences on the central nervous system

Visceral sensations

Sensations associated with the abdominal viscera occur in health and disease. Epigastric fullness and emptiness are equated with satiety and hunger respectively, but how much of these sensations actually arise from the gut or are merely 'referred' to the gut is not clear. Other sensations, such as the degree of fullness and nature of contents (e.g. solid, gas) of the colonorectal region, cue the behaviours related to defaecation and for the release of flatus. Disorders of gut function are indicated by sensations of pain, nausea and bloating. One of the major challenges in this area is understanding the relationship between the stimulus at the gut level and the sensation produced, and this aspect is discussed further below. Sensations of pain from the gut are conveyed by the spinal afferents, whilst the vagal afferents are thought to be involved mainly in signalling non-painful sensations such as emptiness and fullness of the stomach (see Andrews, 1986b; Cervero, 1988; Grundy & Scratchard, 1988 for reviews). The role of the visceral afferents in the genesis of the sensation of nausea is at present unclear. If abnormal motility patterns are associated with nausea, as appears to be the case (e.g. Stern *et al.*, 1987), the visceral afferents are quite capable of signalling these to the CNS and thus contributing to the overall feeling of visceral malaise (see Andrews and Hawthorn, 1988 for further discussion).

Arousal

The mechanism usually implicated in the production of weakness and decreased consciousness associated with rapid gastric emptying involves changes in blood glucose levels, but they could as easily be accounted for by intense visceral afferent activity. Ginzel (1973) demonstrated inhibition of extensor muscle motor reflexes by vagal afferent activation in the cat, and further feline studies have demonstrated the induction of sleep by intestinal and splanchnic and vagal nerve stimulation (Kukorelli & Juhasz, 1976, 1977).

Vasopressin secretion

One further influence that abdominal visceral afferents have on the central nervous system is the release of vasopressin from the posterior pituitary. Stimulation of abdominal vagal afferents and handling of the gut during surgery (Ukai *et al.*, 1968; Hawthorn *et al.*, 1988a) both evoke a substantial release of vasopressin. The function of this large increase in plasma vasopressin is unclear, but the gut muscle, in common with smooth muscle in several other areas, is sensitive to vasopressin and thus it is possible that these high levels of vasopressin may be involved in the genesis of gut motor patterns, e.g. in patients with chronic idiopathic constipation, vasopressin increased the number of propagating spike bursts in the colon and induced defaecation in four out of 10 patients (Schang *et al.*, 1987).

INTRINSIC AFFERENTS

The afferent neurones within the enteric nervous system have many functions which parallel those of extrinsic afferents (Gershon & Erde, 1981; Llewellyn-Smith *et al.*, 1983). Thus in the enteric system there are local reflexes activated by distension of a gut segment, or luminal chemicals which are involved in exocrine (e.g. gastric acid, chloride from the intestinal mucosa) and endocrine (e.g. gastrin) secretions from the gut mucosa, as well as influencing the contractile activity of the muscle, the best example of this being the peristaltic reflex (Costa & Furness, 1976). The reflex effects of intrinsic afferent activation usually tend to be local, although there is growing evidence suggesting that longer intramural neurones may be involved in coordinating activity between regions such as the terminal oesophagus and proximal stomach and the terminal antrum and duodenum (e.g. Ohta *et al.*, 1985).

THE ANATOMY, PHYSIOLOGY AND PHARMACOLOGY OF ABDOMINAL VISCERAL AFFERENTS

Afferent numbers and pathways

Two sets of afferents, extrinsic and intrinsic, are relevant to this review (see Fig. 10.2). The intrinsic afferents are a component of the ENS, contained predominantly in Meissner's and Auerbach's plexuses in the gut wall. In general, whilst a great deal is known of the neurochemistry, morphology and electrophysiological characteristics of the enteric motorneurones and interneurones, the properties of the intrinsic afferents are considerably less well understood (Wood, 1983). Although many of the ideas developed in this review apply to the intrinsic afferent innervation, substantially more is known of the extrinsic afferents and their possible involvement in gastrointestinal disease, and therefore this review will focus on this afferent group, making only passing reference to the intrinsic afferent nerves.

The extrinsic afferent innervation of the gut is provided by afferent axons travelling in the vagus, splanchnic, hypogastric and pelvic nerves. Abdominal vagal afferent axons project to the brainstem, mainly to the subnucleus gelatinosus region of the nucleus tractus solitarius, with a minor projection to the area postrema (for review see Leslie, 1985). The splanchnic, hypogastric and pelvic afferents project to the dorsal horn of the spinal cord (for review see Cervero, 1988). In all non-ruminant species so far investigated, the abdominal vagal trunks have been shown to be 75–90% afferent in composition, with the vast majority of the afferent axons being unmyelinated and hence having conduction velocities <2.5 metres/second. A few hundred small myelinated fibres, thought to be afferent, have been reported to be present in the abdominal vagus of many species. The splanchnic hypogastric and pelvic nerves are probably composed of about 50% afferent fibres overall (calculation for the cat based on data from Jänig & Morrison, 1986; Kuo *et al.*, 1982). In contrast to the vagus, small diameter myelinated fibres (conduction velocity in the A δ range) make a significant contribution with about 25% of the afferents in the greater splanchnic nerve being myelinated. In the cat about 22 000–25 000 afferents supply the abdominal and pelvic viscera but, whilst this appears to be a large number, it has been noted by Cervero (1988) that visceral afferent fibres represent less than 10% of the total afferent inflow to the thoracolumbar spinal cord. The vagus nerve in the cat contains about 27 000 afferents conveying information from the abdominal viscera. These observations from the cat give some impression of the magnitude of the afferent innervation of the gut, but what is known of man? Light and electron microscope studies of the abdominal vagal trunks in man (Mackay & Andrews, 1983) have demonstrated the presence of a large number of unmyelinated fibres and a few myelinated fibres, and this has been confirmed by recording studies of compound action potentials from segments of vagal trunks removed during truncal vagotomy (Andrews & Taylor, 1982). Unfortunately it is impossible to state the afferent : efferent ratio for the abdominal vagus or splanchnic nerves in man, since to obtain such figures it is necessary to compare the number of axons in the nerve trunk in question in intact subjects and in those in which the nerve trunk has been sectioned chronically at a point central to the cell bodies of the afferent axons: the nodose ganglion for the vagus and the dorsal root ganglia for the spinal nerves. Quantitative studies in a range of animals have so far failed to demonstrate a relationship between size of animal (and hence gut size) and vagal afferent number. Unless the vagal afferents branch more extensively in the periphery in larger animals, it is likely that larger (non-ruminant) animals have poorer discrimination of visceral events. In addition, the number of vagal efferents is unrelated to the mass of gut tissue supplied, but this may not have any functional consequences, as the enteric nervous system could be used to disseminate the vagal efferent drive over the required area.

In addition to the vagal and spinal afferents described above, which have been known for many years, more recent studies have identified two other afferent fibre types. Firstly, some afferents in the submucous or myenteric plexuses have axons travelling with the sympathetic nerves which terminate in the coeliac or inferior mesenteric ganglia and synapse with postganglionic sympathetic neurones, making a prevertebral reflex arc. Such reflexes are thought to have an important role in the control of colonic motility (King & Szurszewski, 1984). Secondly, a group of afferents with cell bodies in the gut wall (cf. the more usual type of spinal afferent with cell bodies in the dorsal root ganglia) have axons projecting directly to the spinal cord via the dorsal roots. This type of afferent has so far only been described in a discrete region just proximal to the external anal sphincter in the guinea-pig and, whilst electrophysiological recordings have yet to be made from these fibres, their location suggests that they may be involved in rectoanal reflex mechanisms (Doerffler-Melly & Neuhuber, 1988).

The nature of the information signalled by abdominal visceral afferents

A detailed description of the characteristics of these afferents is outside the scope of this review and this topic has been reviewed recently by several authors (Mei, 1985; Andrews, 1986b; Janig & Morrison, 1986; Cervero, 1988; Grundy & Scratcherd, 1988). In outline, the types of information signalled relate to the following (see Fig. 10.2):

1 The nature of the luminal contents (osmolarity, carbohydrate and amino acid concentration, temperature, the presence of irritants and possibly food consistency). The receptors involved are probably located in the gut mucosa and the majority of studies suggest that the afferents are in the vagus nerve. This group of afferents are usually referred to as 'mucosal chemoreceptors'.

2 The tension in the muscular wall of the gut. The mechano-receptors in the gut wall are described as being 'in series' with the muscle and hence discharge in response to changes in the tension of the gut wall, whether it is induced actively by contraction of the gut muscle or passively by distension or even local compression. This type of information is signalled in the vagus and splanchnic nerves, although in the case of the latter it is often associated with signalling painful levels of distension. Some of the receptors may be located in the serosal layer of the gut wall.

3 Mesenteric tension. Receptors with afferents in the spinal nerves have been described which respond to distortion of the mesentery and its perivascular endings. These receptors may have an important role in painful sensations from the gut, as their discharge is enhanced by stimuli that put tension on the mesentery, such as respiratory movements and gut motility, both of which are known to exacerbate gut pain.

Coding of afferent information

As with other sensory systems, afferent information is signalled in the form of a frequency code, the frequency of discharge in the afferent being related to the intensity of the stimulus activating the afferent. Thus, if one considers a mechanoreceptor in the muscular wall of the colon, the CNS receives information about the presence of contractions, their magnitude, duration and frequency (Blumberg *et al.*, 1983). By collating the discharge from receptors at different locations along the colon, the direction and speed of propagation of the contractions could be derived. When it is remembered that the entire gut from oesophagus to the colon is supplied by afferent fibres, the amount of information signalled relating to gut function must be considerable. In the foregoing section (p. 94) the uses made of this information were discussed, but what determines which action is taken? The answer to this question is not completely known, but we can speculate on the principles involved by considering two examples, one from the stomach and the other from the colon.

Following the entry of a normal-sized meal into the stomach, vagal mechanoreceptors with receptive fields in the gastric body signal the overall level of tension in the gastric wall, which is related to the degree of filling of the stomach (Andrews *et al.*, 1980). The consequence of activation of these afferents is to evoke reflex relaxation of the gastric corpus muscle to facilitate accommodation of further food and to prevent emptying of the recently ingested food. In addition, acid and pepsin secretion are stimulated and the subject may perceive a sensation of pleasant fullness and satiety. If the subject continues eating, then in addition to the reflex effects on motility and secretion the subject may be aware of epigastric discomfort, nausea or even pain, due either to higher levels of stimulation of the same set of afferents or recruitment of afferents only sensitive to stimuli outside the normal range and which, when activated, give rise to painful sensations (e.g. some biliary afferents; see Chapter 9, this volume; Cervero, 1982). The effect of gastric distension in the absence of gastric pathology is illustrated by the studies by Durrans & Taylor (1986) using an intragastric balloon for obesity treatment. A high proportion of subjects have nausea and vomiting over the first 72 hours, subsiding as the stomach accommodates the balloon and the mechanoreceptors are less intensely stimulated. In addition, adrenal catecholamine secretion may be enhanced and some tensing of the abdominal muscles may be apparent. If the subject persists in eating despite these warning signs, the pain and nausea will probably intensify and finally the emetic prodromata (sweating, salivation, antral dysrhythmias and small intestinal retroperistalsis) will be evoked and vomiting will follow. All the actions described above can result from different levels of activation of the same set of afferents and, although we have used the stomach as an example, this scheme could easily apply to other gut regions. We have described overeating as the cause of more and more intense activation of the afferents to produce a range of effects, but it is easy to see the consequences for a patient in whom the gastric afferents have had their sensitivity altered (Fig. 10.3). This is discussed below (p. 112) with reference to the genesis of anorexia nervosa.

Studies on the effects of colorectal distension on pseudoaffective

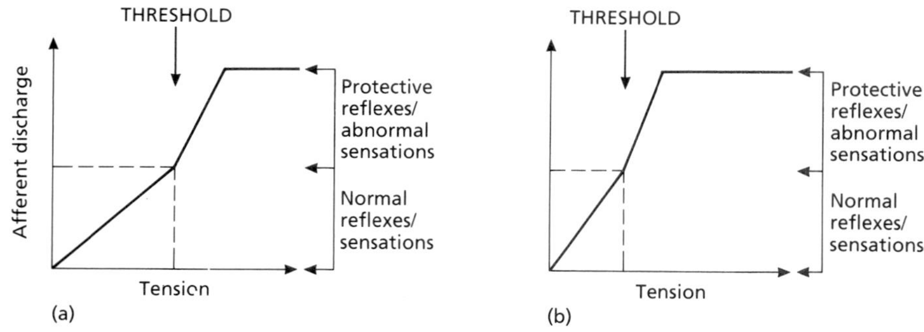

Fig. 10.3. Diagram illustrating the effects of sensitization of a mechanoreceptive afferent on the afferent discharge and the reflex consequences. (a) As the tension in the muscle increases, the afferent discharge also increases, giving rise to normal gut motor reflexes involved in digestion. With increased stimulation a 'threshold' level is exceeded, above which protective reflexes (e.g. vomiting) and abnormal sensations (pain) are evoked. (b) If the afferent is sensitized, the 'threshold' will be reached at a lower level of stimulation; in consequence the 'normal' levels of mechanoreceptor stimulation will give rise to 'abnormal' reflex responses. Note that this could also occur if the length–tension properties of the muscle were altered rather than the sensitivity of the afferent modified.

reflexes (e.g. changes in blood pressure, abdominal muscle tensing)
in the conscious rat give important insights into some of the
mechanisms that may be involved in colonic disease. Low level
distension (13.2 ± 0.7 mmHg) produced reflex relaxation of the
anal sphincters (i.e. defaecation is triggered). Further distension
evoked a graded increase in blood pressure and heart rate and when
the distending pressure reached 22.4 ± 0.9 mmHg abdominal and
hindlimb muscle contraction occurred, indicative of a nociceptive
response (Ness & Gebhart, 1988a). Taking these results together
with the electrophysiological characteristics of colonic afferents
(Blumberg et al., 1983; Ness & Gebhart, 1987, 1988b), it can be
seen that the motor responses evoked are closely related to features
of the afferent signal and hence if that signal is perturbed then the
evoked motor activity is likely to be perturbed. This is discussed
further (p. 107) in relation to colonic disease.

Afferent receptor structure

In contrast to many other types of receptor (e.g. Meissner's corpuscles, Merkel's discs, rods and cones, taste buds, carotid bodies),
relatively little is known of the structure of the receptor elements
involved in the detection of events in the abdominal viscera (see
Neuhuber, 1987 and Grundy, 1988 for a discussion of this topic).
Mechanoreceptive afferents terminate in the muscular layers of the
gut wall as a tapering extension of an unmyelinated axon. Whilst
no specialized receptor structure analogous to muscle spindles or
Pacinian corpuscles has been identified, the termination of the
axon is specialized for the transformation and transduction of the
mechanical event into a series of impulses in the afferent axon. The
visceral afferents responsible for signalling aspects of the luminal
environment, the so-called chemoreceptors (see p. 100, appear to
have a specialized receptor structure, although studies of this aspect
of visceral afferents is probably the one that has been least investigated. It has been proposed by several authors (e.g. Mei, 1985)
that the anatomical substrate for the mucosal chemoreceptor is a
mucosal cell which, when activated by an appropriate stimulus
in the lumen, releases a neuroactive agent from its basal surface
to evoke a discharge in an afferent axon terminating in close
proximity. Some anatomical evidence in support of this idea comes
from anatomical studies by Newson et al. (1982), which showed
vagal afferent axons terminating in the basal lamina of the small
intestine of the cat, in close proximity to enterochromaffin cells
and cells they termed 'taste cells'. Studies in the stomach have
identified vagal afferents terminating as free endings near the
mucous membrane (Sato & Koyano, 1987), although it is not yet
clear whether they terminate in relation to any particular mucosal
cell type (e.g. enterochromaffin cells, mast cells). Further support

for this anatomical arrangement representing a chemoreceptor comes from other chemoreceptor systems such as the taste buds, arterial chemoreceptors and airway irritant receptors, all of which have this type of organization (Barlow & Mollon, 1982; Pack & Widdicombe, 1984). It must be emphasized that this structure for the chemoreceptors in the gut is still speculative and need not be the basis of all chemoreception in the gut. Chemicals in the lumen could gain access to the afferent axons in the basal lamina via the intercellular junctions and activate them directly. Whilst entero-chromaffin cells releasing 5HT onto afferents could account for the structural basis of chemoreceptors in the duodenum where mucosal 5HT levels are high (Ahlman & Dahlstrom, 1983), regions such as the stomach where mucosal 5HT is sparse would presumably employ other mucosally stored agents such as gastrin to activate the afferents. It is clearly important to understand the structure of the chemoreceptors since, if the scheme outlined above is the correct one, identification of the mucosal agents involved in afferent activation could lead to the development of a range of drugs to modify chemoreceptor activity in different gut regions. Some progress has been made in this direction and is discussed in the section on the pharmacology of visceral afferents below.

The pharmacology of gut afferents

This section examines the responses of the visceral afferents to a variety of chemicals, either injected into the arterial supply to the organ from which the afferent originates or applied topically to the gut in the region of the afferents' receptive field. The fact that many visceral afferents respond to a range of chemicals has implications for understanding the nature of the transduction process, the regulation of afferent sensitivity and the design of novel drug therapy. Gut mechanoreceptors with afferent fibres in the vagus nerve in various species have been reported to be activated by the following agents: 5HT; 2-methyl-5HT and phenylbiguanide ($5HT_3$ receptor agonists); nicotine; adrenaline; pentagastrin; insulin; prostaglandin; bradykinin; CCK-8; and veratridine and lobeline (plant alkaloids) (Paintal, 1954; Douglas & Ritchie, 1957; Paintal, 1964; Cottrell & Iggo, 1984a; Clarke & Davison, 1988; Andrews & Davidson, 1990). One problem in dealing with mechanoreceptors is that most of the above agents induce contraction of gut muscle and hence would be expected to induce activation by this mechanism alone. However, whilst there is debate over the extent to which the discharge is secondary to contraction (e.g. see Cottrell & Iggo, 1984a, 1984b), most authors agree that at least a component of the response, with some of these agents, is due to a direct effect on the afferent ending. Too few studies have been undertaken on vagal mucosal afferents to draw any firm conclusions, although our own studies in the ferret have shown that gastric mucosal chemoreceptors can be activated by 5HT (Davidson & Andrews, 1988).

The chemosensitivity of the splanchnic afferents has been investigated primarily from the aspect of understanding the mechanism by which pain is induced by tissue damage. Afferents in the stomach, small and large intestine respond to bradykinin, 5HT and substance P and, as with the vagal mechanoreceptors, muscle contractions account for some but not all responses (Haupt *et al.*, 1983; Longhurst *et al.*, 1984b; Lew & Longhurst, 1986).

The major conclusion that can be drawn from these studies is that the gut afferents can be influenced by a variety of endogenous agents. These agents may be involved in the normal transduction process in mucosal chemoreceptors (see above), or could modify the sensitivity of the afferents to their natural stimuli, and it is this aspect that is the subject of the next section.

Control of afferent sensitivity

The sensitivity of an afferent is taken to mean the number of action potentials occurring in the afferent fibre in response to a given stimulus in a healthy subject. Hence an increase in sensitivity results in a greater discharge for the same intensity of stimulus or, in the case of afferents that usually respond only to high intensity stimuli, their threshold is reduced. To deal fully with the role of visceral afferents in gut disease this definition needs to be extended to incorporate the factors influencing the central processing of visceral afferent information. A detailed discussion of the central processing of visceral afferent information from the gut is outside the scope of this chapter and the topic has been reviewed by Andrews (1986b) and Cervero (1988) (see also Chapter 9). The main point of relevance to this chapter is that a number of mechanisms exist in the brainstem and spinal cord that can enhance or suppress the afferent signal originating from the gut. The most relevant here are those modifying the transmission of nociceptive information, a defect which may be manifested as a change in visceral pain sensitivity such as appears to occur in some gastrointestinal disorders. The remainder of this section deals with the factors involved in the regulation of afferent sensitivity at a peripheral site in the gut wall.

The sensitivity of mechanoreceptors in the gut wall will depend to a large extent upon the prevailing tension in the gut wall. When the resting tension is high, the resting discharge in the afferent will be higher than if the muscle was in a relaxed state. In response to the same distending stimulus, the final discharge will be higher in the tissue with the higher resting tension because the final tension achieved is higher. The practical implication of this is that if a tissue develops an abnormally high resting tension (for example because of elevated activity in cholinergic excitatory nerves, decreased activity in non-adrenergic non-cholinergic inhibitory systems, or raised motilin levels) when the tissue becomes stretched by food or faeces, the mechanoreceptor discharge may reach higher than normal levels and produce particularly unpleasant sensations.

The second factor implicated in regulating the sensitivity of afferents involves the action of endogenous or exogenous chemicals on the afferent axons. As yet very few electrophysiological studies have been undertaken to investigate directly changes in the sensitivity of gastrointestinal afferents (but see Chapter 9), and therefore the mechanisms likely to be operating in the gut will be discussed by reference to more detailed studies in other sensory systems. In Japan, subacute myelo-optic neuropathy (SMON) was found to be associated with the ingestion of clioquinol (Sobue, 1979). The symptoms caused by this agent include abdominal fullness, constipation and intense abdominal pain. Electrophysiological studies of testicular polymodal receptors revealed that whilst clioquinol had little effect on the afferent discharge in its own right, it did however produce a marked sensitization of the afferents to other stimuli (Kumazawa & Mizumura, 1984). It is therefore likely that the abdominal reactions to clioquinol are due to sensitization of gut afferents. A further example of afferent sensitization comes from studies of slowly conducting afferents in joints, skin and skeletal muscles. Using carageenin to inflame the tissues, it has been demonstrated that the afferents in inflamed tissue have a higher resting discharge and a lowered threshold to mechanical stimulation (Coggeshall *et al.*, 1983; Schaible & Schmidt, 1985; Kocher *et al.*, 1987; Berberich *et al.*, 1988). These agents probably sensitize the afferents by causing the release of endogenous agents which then act on the afferents to modify their characteristics. When a tissue becomes inflamed a number of neuroactive agents are released including 5HT, prostaglandin and bradykinin, all of which have been demonstrated electrophysiologically to enhance the sensitivity of afferents in a number of systems (e.g. Sicuteri, 1968; Beck & Handwerker, 1974; Mense, 1981). Although we do not yet have comparable studies in the gut, it would be surprising if similar mechanisms were not operating, in view of the similarities in the electrophysiological and pharmacological characteristics of some of the afferents described above and some of the more polymodal gut afferents, and the presence in the gut wall of agents known to influence the sensitivity of afferents.

EVIDENCE FOR THE INVOLVEMENT OF AFFERENTS IN GASTROINTESTINAL DISEASE

One of the problems in attempting to assess the role of disturbed visceral afferent function in gastrointestinal disease is that very few studies have directly investigated this problem. The dicussion below examines some of the studies which are suggestive of an involvement of modified afferent activity in the various gut disorders. From the foregoing discussion it can be seen that afferents may be involved in three main ways:

1 An afferent may have its sensitivity enhanced or decreased by factors acting at either a peripheral or a central site.

2 An afferent may be involved in signalling abnormal activity occurring in the organ (e.g. overdistension) and hence giving rise to visceral sensations associated with gut disease (e.g. pain, bloating).

3 An afferent may be the detector of a toxin in the gut lumen or circulation and evoke the visceral and somatic components of the vomiting reflex to rid the body of the toxin.

The examples discussed below illustrate these various types of involvement of visceral afferents in a number of clinical situations, all of which may be amenable to therapy directed at modifying afferent transmission.

Irritable bowel syndrome and pain

The difficulty of identifying the afferent (either at its peripheral terminal or central projection) as the site of the disorder is best illustrated by reference to a simple example relating to one of the more common symptoms of IBS, that of lower bowel pain a few hours after a meal, associated with the entry of digested food into the colon as indicated by breath hydrogen concentration (Cann & Read, 1985). Two mechanisms which account for this observation are discussed below and are illustrated in Fig. 10.3).

In some IBS patients the amplitude of colonic pressure waves (measured over a 100 minute period) following a 1000 kcal meal was greater than in controls (Rogers et al., 1989). Possibly the ability of the colonic muscle to relax may be impaired, causing an abnormally large increase in colonic wall tension when the colon is distended. As the mechanoreceptors in the muscular wall of the gut discharge in response to contraction and distension of the muscle, either response to digested food will evoke a discharge. In addition, mechanoreceptors in the colon discharge in response to local ischaemia which could be induced by large contractions (Haupt et al., 1983). In healthy subjects it is known that high levels of colonic distension or large contractions evoke pain (Lipkin & Sleisenger, 1958). Thus it might logically be concluded that the pain of IBS is due to an inappropriate response of the muscle to digested food, leading to a high level afferent discharge sufficient to evoke a sensation of pain, or to the recruitment of specific high threshold nociceptors such as those described in the gall bladder (Cervero, 1982). The prime lesion in such cases could be the enteric non-adrenergic, non-cholinergic inhibitory nerves or the extrinsic nerves influencing them. It is worth noting here that factors other than

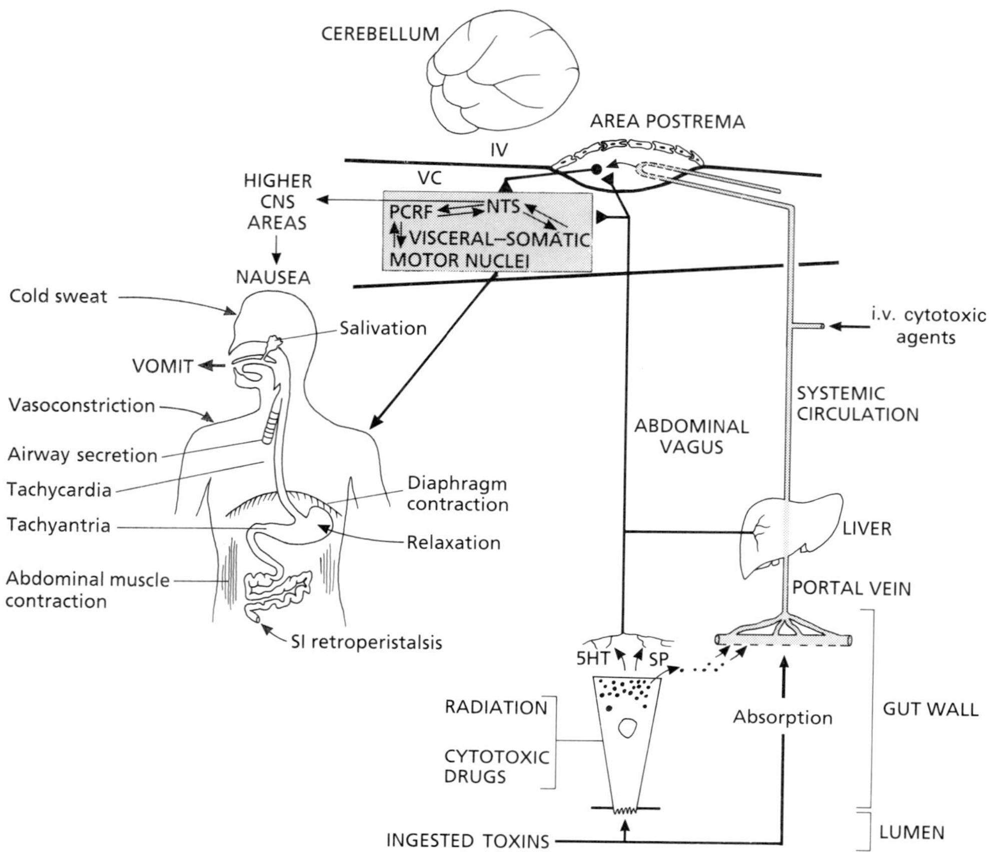

Fig. 10.4. A summary of the major components of the vomiting reflex. The left of the figure shows the visceral and somatic motor components of the reflex that are coordinated by the 'vomiting centre' (VC), represented by the interactions between the visceral and somatic motor nuclei, the parvicellular reticular formation (PCRF) and the nucleus tractus solitarius (NTS). It is proposed that, in addition to agents acting on the area postrema via the circulation, vomiting can also be evoked by activation of abdominal vagal afferents. It is envisaged that these afferents are activated or sensitized by 5HT or other agents released by luminal or systemic emetic stimuli. IV = fourth ventricle; SP = substance P; SI = small intestine. (Redrawn with permission from Andrews *et al.*, 1988.)

distending volume *per se* are involved in the genesis of gut pain. In the colon it has been shown that the duration of distension also influences the response, with high levels of distension eliciting a report of pain in a few seconds whereas lower levels are only perceived as painful after a delay, with the report of pain often being preceded by a sensation of pressure (Lipkin & Sleisenger, 1958). Other distension studies have demonstrated that the length of bowel distended is also a significant factor (Lewis, 1942).

An equally valid but less often considered mechanism does not rely on a defect in the motor response of the colon but is based on a modification of afferent function. Sensations from the gut, as with other sensory systems, are generated as a result of a particular spatio-temporal discharge in a set of afferents originating from a particular structure with which the perceived sensation is associated. Irrespective of how the discharge is evoked, if it is of the right frequency, duration and pattern a sensation will be perceived. If we consider the colon, then to produce pain in response to the presence of digested food all that is required is for the sensitivity of the colonic afferent mechanoreceptors to be increased, so that normal levels of distension or contraction evoke a discharge that would usually only be produced by abnormal levels of distension or contraction. The site of sensitization of the mechanoreceptors may be in the gut wall, the spinal cord (see p. 105) or in the supraspinal mechanisms that modulate the transmission of afferent traffic in the spinal cord (see Cervero, 1988). The foregoing discussion has focused on a role for the mechanoreceptors, but this is not meant to suggest that mucosal chemoreceptors are not involved. Clinical studies with the diphenolic laxative bisacodyl show that, apart from its direct stimulant effects on motility when applied to the colonic mucosa, it sensitizes the mucosa so that even saline applied to the mucosa will stimulate activity (Hardcastle & Mann, 1968). Studies in the rat colon have shown bisacodyl stimulates the release of prostaglandin E (Beubler & Juan, 1978). Since prostaglandins can sensitize afferents, it may be that mucosal prostaglandins are involved in regulation of colonic afferent sensitivity. Serotonin is also found in large quantities in colonic mucosa (Resnick & Gray, 1961) and can sensitize afferents (see p. 105).

It is obviously important to distinguish between these two different mechanisms outlined above, since they require different therapeutic approaches, but how can this be done? In animal studies it is relatively simple to record the discharge in afferent fibres and to test the effects of stimulation before and after giving agents which sensitize the afferents. This approach has been used in a number of afferent systems but studies in the gut are in their infancy. One of the problems is that, whilst such studies give insights into the regulation of afferent sensitivity, it is not possible to study the afferent changes actually occurring in the disease because there is no accepted animal model of IBS. It may be possible in clinical studies to distinguish between the above mechanisms, using carefully controlled inflation studies similar to those reported by Richter *et al.* (1986) in their studies of non-cardiac chest pain in man. By measuring pressure/volume relationships in the oesophagus, they were able to conclude that in some patients pain was induced at a lower level of inflation than controls, even though the pressure/volume relationships were similar in both groups. The conclusion from this study is that, although these patients have a lower pain threshold, it is not due to an abnormal motor response to the distensive stimulus, but may be due to either sensitization of afferents at a peripheral site or a change in central processing of the afferent signal. In IBS patients some authors have reported a lower pain threshold to colonic distension (Ritchie, 1985) and, whilst this is consistent with a mechanism involving the afferents, in the absence of data showing colonic pressure/volume relationships no firmer conclusion can be drawn. In an earlier study, Latimer *et al.* (1979) were unable to demonstrate a difference in the pain response to distension of the sigmoid colon between normal subjects, IBS patients and psychoneurotic patients without bowel symptoms.

It must be emphasized that the mechanisms above represent two extremes of a spectrum and it is of course possible that both operate to different degrees in different patients. Also it is likely that even if the prime lesion is in the afferents this will lead to abnormal reflex motor patterns, and therefore in clinical studies alone it may be impossible to identify the relative contribution of each to the overall clinical picture.

In IBS some authors report disorders of micturition including frequency, urgency and hesitancy (see Chapter 5). Colonic afferents in the pelvic nerve can inhibit spontaneous bladder motility, reduce activity in vesicle efferent nerves and increase the micturition threshold (Floyd *et al.*, 1982). Thus there is little doubt that the colon can influence bladder function, and this raises the possibility that some of the disorders of micturition seen in some cases of IBS may be secondary to a colonic motor or afferent disorder, rather than further manifestations of a more general pelvic neuropathy. The back pain occurring in IBS can be accounted for by viscerosomatic convergence between colonic and cutaneous afferents in the spinal cord (Ness & Gebhart, 1988a,b), as is the case for other types of referred visceral pain (Cervero 1988).

One of the puzzling aspects of IBS is why it is so much more common in females. There is no obvious explanation, but since female sex hormones have effects on gastrointestinal smooth muscle this may be a contributing factor. An additional possible involvement of sex hormones comes from studies showing that, in the uterus of guinea-pigs and women, the levels of adrenergic neurotransmitters and their synthesizing enzymes decrease dramatically during pregnancy, indicating degeneration of the short adrenergic neurones supplying the myometrium (Thorbert *et al.*, 1978, 1979). Is it possible that sex hormones could under some circumstances cause a deletion of neurones from other pelvic structures such as the colon? If a deletion of neurones occurs, it must be confined to inhibitory neurones involved in relaxation of the colon, so that colonic wall tension and contraction amplitude are increased, giving rise to the effects on afferents described on pp. 107–108.

Visceral afferents have at least two types of involvement in the pathophysiology of peptic ulceration. First, the splanchnic afferents are the pathway by which the painful sensations from the ulcer reach the CNS. The actual cause of the pain is still not known. Recent studies investigating the reproducibility of duodenal ulcer pain by acid in symptomatic and non-symptomatic patients showed that acid induced pain in 42% of symptomatic and 13% of asymptomatic subjects (Kang *et al.*, 1989). These results suggest that in the symptomatic subjects the ulcer crater is more sensitive to acid and implicates local agents released in the vicinity of the ulcer in influencing the sensitivity of the afferent. Studies by Wolf (1965) on his fistulated subject Tom demonstrated that pinching or faradic stimulation of the normal gastic mucosa did not evoke pain, but after the mucosa was made oedematous and inflamed (using 1 N HCl and powdered mustard!) the same stimuli were painful. Although this study is rather crude, it does demonstrate dramatically how the state of the mucosa can influence the sensations produced in response to a particular stimulus. It would be of interest to see how far from the crater of a peptic ulcer the region of heightened sensitivity extends, and the nature of chemical changes occurring in the mucosa in these regions. Adenosine or related compounds may be involved, as systemic adenosine can mimic ulcer pain in duodenal ulcer patients (Watt *et al.*, 1987) and lysed erythrocytes evoke pain, at least in part because of release of adenosine compounds (Higashi, 1986). If the nature of the chemical changes occurring in the ulcer crater was known, some attempt could be made to block the effect of these agents on the splanchnic afferents and help to alleviate the pain.

The second involvement of afferents in ulcers is a rather speculative one and is based solely on animal studies. In rats given the neurotoxin capsaicin at birth to destroy unmyelinated visceral afferents, gastric lesions induced by indomethacin, ethanol or cysteamine were larger than in control animals (Holzer & Sametz, 1986). One conclusion from this study is that afferents are involved to some degree in gastric mucosal protection, possibly by means of the axon reflexes described on p. 96. On the basis of this preliminary evidence one might suggest that in some gastric ulcer patients this pathway is defective and could be activated by agonist drugs acting on the afferent terminals.

DISORDERS OF DEFAECATION

The defaecation reflex consists of a spinal reflex activated by the presence of faecal material in the colonorectal region but which can be enhanced or suppressed by supraspinal structures. Defects in afferents in the colonorectal region may be involved in disorders of defaecation in the following way. At a particular colonorectal distending volume, the urge to defaecate is perceived and, if socially convenient, the reflex is reinforced by supraspinal influences and defaecation will ensue. If however the afferents have a blunted response, then faecal material will build up until the threshold is reached (the delay being related to the degree of afferent impairment) when defaecation will occur, but it may not be complete. Thus it is possible for a residue of faeces to accumulate, leading to distension-induced damage to the muscle and further contributing to the constipation due to the original afferent lesion. In patients with sensitized afferents or with a high colonorectal muscle tone, the defaecation reflex will be triggered at smaller volumes. The effect of this is unlikely to be diarrhoea but will probably be the passing of larger numbers of smaller stools, with perhaps little if any effect on total stool weight.

INTESTINAL TRANSPORT

The intestinal secretory response to toxic agents such as cholera toxin requires the integrity of the enteric nerves, and some authors have proposed a model in which 5HT is released by the toxin from the enterochromaffin cell and activates a local intramural afferent neurone, which in turn elicits the secretory response in the enterocyte (Jodal & Lundgren, 1987). Blockade of the activation of the intramural afferent by a 5HT receptor antagonist could provide a novel method for alleviating diarrhoea induced by luminal agents acting via this pathway, possibly including the types of diarrhoea induced by some foods in sensitized individuals. Studies by Cuthbert (Chapter 13 this volume; Baird & Cuthbert, 1987) indicate that the $5HT_3$ receptor antagonist ICS-205-930 markedly reduces the intestinal chloride secretory response to 5HT and β-lactoglobulin in cow-milk-sensitized guinea-pig. The mechanisms outlined above could equally well apply to the disruption of motility induced by bacterial or viral agents.

DISORDERS OF FOOD INTAKE

There is growing evidence that in some cases primary anorexia nervosa may be successfully treated by gastrokinetic agents, the implication being that a gastric motility disorder is involved in the genesis of the changes in food intake. How could this occur? Activation of afferent nerves from the stomach is responsible for the initial postprandial phase of satiety, with the vagus playing the major role. Satiety is associated with a pleasant sensation of epigastric fullness, which subsides as the food is emptied from the

stomach and other satiety signals begin to operate. If the afferents
from the stomach are activated further due to excessive distension
of the stomach by overeating, or by the accumulation of food and
secretions in a subject with gastric stasis, then sensations of nausea,
bloating and pain result (see p. 101 for further discussion of mechanism). Slowing of gastric emptying is capable of decreasing food
intake in rats, and it is this gastric effect that probably accounts for
at least some of the suppressant effects of fenfluramine on food
intake (Booth *et al.*, 1986).

Nausea and pain represent two of the most potent aversive
stimuli and, contrary to popular belief, nausea is the more strongly
aversive in man (Pelchat & Rozin, 1982). Thus it is possible that
the genesis of anorexia nervosa involves the development of a
learned aversion, such that food intake is decreased to avoid
the nausea and pain that results from its intake. As food intake
decreases the stomach will 'shrink' as it does in severe dieting, with
the result that when it is distended with a smaller volume the
resulting wall tension is higher, causing the afferent discharge to be
elevated (see p. 108). If slowed gastric emptying is the original
cause, a gastrokinetic will help to break the cycle provided the
subject can be persuaded to eat. This may not be as easy as it
appears, as even a single exposure to a food that causes nausea can
result in refusal of that food for the rest of one's life (Pelchat &
Rozin, 1982).

In some patients the starting point for a decrease in food intake
could be the sensitization of gastric afferents, such that nausea or
pain are evoked at conventional meal sizes. Studies in the rat
implicate CCK-8 in the activation of afferents in the gut wall as
being involved in the postprandial satiety signal. An antagonist to
peripheral CCK-8 receptors (L364–718) antagonized the reduction
of food intake produced by CCK-8 and increased the intake of
palatable food in non-deprived rats (Hewson *et al.*, 1988).

These studies suggest that agonist drugs acting on afferents in the
gut wall may be of use in the treatment of obesity by giving a false
satiety signal, and antagonists may be helpful in anorexia nervosa
and other diseases where food ingestion results in unpleasant
sensations or vomiting by blunting the afferent signal.

VOMITING

The introduction of $5HT_3$ receptor antagonists such as Kytril and
Zofran has revolutionized the treatment of vomiting induced by
cancer chemotherapeutic drugs. The site and mechanism of action
of the $5HT_3$ receptor antagonists and chemotherapeutic agents is
not known with certainty, but a model that accounts for many (but
not all) of the experimental observations has been proposed by
Andrews *et al.* (1988) and is shown in Fig. 10.4. In this model it is

proposed that the cytotoxic drugs evoke the release of 5HT from the gut enterochromaffin cells, and that this either directly activates the vagal afferents or sensitizes them to other agents (see p. 105). One site of action of the $5HT_3$ receptor antagonists is within the gut wall on the vagal afferent terminals, but an additional central site cannot be excluded particularly in view of studies demonstrating binding sites for $5HT_3$ receptor ligands in the area postrema (Barnes *et al.*, 1988). It must be emphasized that these agents are not universal antiemetics (they have no effect on apomorphine or motion-induced vomiting) but will only be effective in systems where $5HT_3$ receptors are activated. Examples where this may be the case are the nausea and vomiting associated with rapid gastric emptying (Drapanas *et al.*, 1962) or diseases in which the intestinal mucosa becomes damaged or inflamed (e.g. by infection), leading to the local release of 5HT. It is debatable whether vomiting induced purely by activation of mechanoreceptors rather than mucosal chemoreceptors will be affected by this class of agents (but see Moss and Sanger, 1987). In addition the gut region on which the emetic stimulus is acting may be important, as it is unlikely that 5HT is involved in afferent activation in all regions of the gut.

THERAPEUTIC APPROACHES TO THE MODIFICATION OF AFFERENT ACTIVITY

This section summarizes some of the therapeutic approaches discussed at various points in the text and outlines others that may be adapted for use in gut disorders.

Blockade of receptors at the peripheral afferent terminals

This approach relies on identification of the locally released agents that cause activation of the afferents. The best current examples in the gut appear to be the CCK-8 and $5HT_3$ receptor antagonists. Agents acting on the afferents may be of use in a variety of gut-related disorders including food intake, some forms of vomiting and diarrhoea, gut pain and defaecation problems. Some suggestion for the involvement of $5HT_3$ receptors in gut pain comes from the studies of Moss and Sanger (1987), showing that cardiovascular response to gut distension (one of the pseudoaffective responses) are reduced in the rat by the $5HT_3$ receptor antagonist Kytril. An additional site of action in the spinal cord cannot be excluded, as $5HT_3$ receptors have been implicated in the spinal nociceptive pathway (Glaum *et al.*, 1988). In order to identify agents for clinical use, it will be necessary to study the activation of afferent nerves in both normal and diseased tissue, in view of the complex chemical transformations occurring when tissue is inflamed or damaged. This approach is well illustrated by studies demonstrating inhibition of the discharge in afferents originating in the inflamed knee joint by opiates acting at a peripheral site (Russell *et al.*, 1987).

Activation of receptors at peripheral afferent terminals

No clinical examples exist of this approach, with the possible exception of bisacodyl (see p. 109), but agents that activate or even sensitize afferents may have some use in activating reflexes in a gut with ileus or in providing an artificial satiety signal in the treatment of obesity. In addition we have seen that vagal afferents may be involved in cytoprotection, possibly via axon reflexes (see p. 96). Activation of these reflexes may give another approach to ulcer therapy.

Blockade of action potential generation in afferents

If it is not possible to block the binding of the endogenous agonist to the afferent axon, can action potential be blocked by interfering with the cellular events intervening between the two events? Studies by Dray *et al.* (1988) in cutaneous nociceptors have shown that bradykinin acts via the activation of protein kinase C, an enzyme that is known to be involved in the regulation of calcium, potassium and chloride channels (Kaczmarek, 1987). This raises the possibility of using inhibitors of protein kinase C (e.g. staurosporine) as antinociceptive agents, and illustrates the general principle of using agents interfering with intracellular mechanisms as a means of modifying afferent activity. The production of the action potential could also be influenced by using agents that block the ion channels in the afferent axon or its generator region (cf. verapamil on smooth muscle).

Modification of the release of local mediators

The release of local mediators in response to damage of the gut wall appears to be a significant factor in sensitizing or activating afferents, and hence blockade of this release may offer another approach in the treatment of some gut disorders. Two cells are likely to be involved, the mast cell and the enterochromaffin cell (see Chapters 13 & 14). The regulation of the release of mediators from mast cells has been reviewed in Chapter 14 this volume, therefore this discussion will be confined to enterochromaffin cells. In addition to local luminal influences, the release of 5HT is modulated by cholinergic and β-adrenergic receptors, and it may be possible to exploit these to minimize the release of 5HT or other mucosal agents during tissue damage (Pairet *et al.*, 1986; Petterson, 1979).

The afferents from the gut project to the medulla and spinal cord and blockade of transmission at these sites could be used to modify visceral sensation and the activation of visceral reflexes. The design of antagonists acting at these sites relies on a knowledge of the neurotransmitters used by the primary afferents. Neurochemical studies have implicated substance P, 5HT, CCK-8, enkephalin and acetylcholine as the major contenders (Leslie, 1985), but so far there have been few attempts to block transmission selectively in the visceral afferent pathways using receptor antagonists to these transmitters. An additional means of modifying central transmission is the use of agents to deplete central neurones of particular neurotransmitters, an example of this approach being anorectal drugs like fenfluramine, which act in part by modifying brain 5HT levels by blocking re-uptake of 5HT into presynaptic neurones (Garattini *et al.*, 1986).

ACKNOWLEDGEMENTS

I wish to thank Dr G. Sanger (Beecham Pharmaceuticals) for his constructive comments on the manuscript and for provocative discussions of this topic. I am grateful to Beecham Pharmaceuticals, Glaxo Group Research and Janssen Pharmaceutical for funding several aspects of the work discussed in this review.

REFERENCES

Abrahamsson, H. & Thoren, P. (1973) Vomiting and reflex vagal relaxation of the stomach elicited from heart receptors in the cat. *Acta Physiol Scand* **88**, 433–439.

Ahlman, H. & Dahlstrom, A. (1983) Vagal mechanisms controlling serotonin release from the gastrointestinal tract and pyloric motor function. In Kral, J.G., Powley, T.L. & Brooks, C.Mc.C. (eds), *Vagal Nerve Function: Behavioural and Methodological Considerations*, pp. 119–140. Elsevier, Amsterdam.

Ahlman, H., Bhargava, H.N., Donahue, P.E., Newson, B., Das Gupta, T.K. & Nyhus, L.M. (1978) The vagal release of 5HT from enterochromaffin cells in the cat. *Acta Physiol Scand* **104**, 262–270.

Andrews, P.L.R. (1986a) The non-adrenergic non-cholinergic innervation of the stomach. *Arch Int Pharmacodyn* **280** (Suppl), 84–109.

Andrews, P.L.R. (1986b) Vagal afferent innervation of the gastrointestinal tract. *Prog Brain Res* **67**, 65–86.

Andrews, P.L.R. & Davidson, H.I.M. (1990) Activation of vagal afferent terminals by 5-hydroxytryptamine is mediated by the 5HT$_3$ receptor in the anaesthetized ferret. *J Physiol* **422**, 928.

Andrews, P.L.R. & Hawthorn, J. (1987) Evidence for an extra-abdominal site of action for the 5HT$_3$ receptor antagonist BRL24924 in the inhibition of radiation-evoked emesis in the ferret. *Neuropharmacology* **26**, 1367–1370.

Andrews, P.L.R. & Hawthorn, J. (1988) The neurophysiology of vomiting. In Read, N.J. & Grundy, D. (eds), *Baillière's Clinical Gastroenterology 2. Neurophysiology of the Gut*, pp. 141–168. Baillière Tindall, London.

Andrews, P.L.R. & Lawes, I.N.C. (1984) Interactions between splanchnic and vagus nerves in the control of mean intragastric pressure in the ferret. *J Physiol* **351**, 473–490.

Andrews, P.L.R & Taylor, T.V. (1982) An electrophysiological study of the posterior abdominal vagus nerve in man. *Clin Sci* **63**, 169–173.

Andrews, P.L.R. & Wood, K.L. (1986) Systemic baclofen stimulates gastric motility and secretion via a central action in the rat. *Br J Pharmac* **89**, 461–467.

Andrews, P.L.R. & Wood, K.L. (1988) Vagally mediated gastric motor and emetic reflexes evoked by stimulation of the antral mucosa in anaesthetized ferrets. *J Physiol* **395**, 1–16.

Andrews, P.L.R., Grundy, D. & Scratcherd, T. (1980) The reflex activation of antral motility by gastric distension in the ferret. *J Physiol* **298**, 79–84.

Andrews, P.L.R., Rapeport, W.G. & Sanger, G.J. (1988) Neuropharmacology of emesis induced by anti-cancer therapy. *Trends Pharmacol Sci* **9**, 334–341.

Baird, A.W. & Cuthbert, A.W. (1987) Neuronal involvement in type I hypersensitivity reactions in gut epithelia. *Br J Pharmacol* **92**, 647–655.

Barlow, H.B. & Mollon, J.D. (1982) *Cambridge Texts in the Physiological Sciences. The Senses*, p. 490. Cambridge University Press, Cambridge.

Barnes, N.M., Costall, B., Naylor, R.J. & Tattersall, F.D. (1988) Identification of $5HT_3$ recognition sites in the ferret area postrema. *J Pharm Pharmacol* **40**.

Beck, P.W. & Handwerker, H.O. (1974) Bradykinin and serotonin effects on various types of cutaneous nerve fibres. *Pflügers Arch* **347**, 209–222.

Berberich, P., Hoheisel, V. & Mense, S., (1988) Effects of carageenin-induced myosites on the discharge properties of group III and IV muscle receptors in the cat. *J Neurophysiol* **59**, 1395–1409.

Bermudez, J., Boyle, E.A., Miner, W.D. & Sanger, G.J. (1988) The anti-emetic potential of the 5-hydroxytryptamine receptor antagonist BRL43694. *Br J Cancer* **58**, 644–650.

Beubler, E. & Juan, H. (1978) Is the effect of diphenolic laxatives mediated via release of prostaglandin E? *Experientia* **34**, 386–387.

Blumberg, H., Haupt, P., Jänig, W. & Kohler, W. (1983) Encoding of visceral noxious stimuli in the discharge patterns of visceral afferent fibres from the colon. *Pflügers Arch* **398**, 33–40.

Booth, D.A., Gibson, E.L. & Baker, B.J. (1986) Gastromotor mechanism of fenfluramine a rexia. In Nicolaidis, S. (ed), *Serotonergic System, Feeding and Body Weight Regulation*, pp. 71–84. Academic Press, London.

Cann, P.A. & Read, N.W. (1985) A disease of the whole gut? In N.W. Read (ed), *Irritable Bowel Syndrome*, pp. 53–63. Grune and Stratton, London.

Cervero, F. (1982) Afferent activity evoked by natural stimulation of the biliary system in the ferret. *Pain* **13**, 137–151.

Cervero, F. (1988) Neurophysiology of gastrointestinal pain. In Read, N.J. & Grundy, D. (eds), *Baillière's Clinical Gastroenterology 2. Neurophysiology of the Gut*, pp. 183–199. Baillière Tindall, London.

Clarke, G.D. & Davidson, J.S. (1988) Mechanical properties and sensitivity to CCK of vagal gastric slowly adapting mechanoreceptors. *Am J Physiol* **255**, G55–61.

Coggeshall, R.E., Hong, K.A.P., Langford, L.A., Schaible, H.G. & Schmidt, R.F. (1983) Discharge characteristics of fine medial articular afferents at rest and during passive movements of inflamed knee joints. *Brain Res* **272**, 185–188.

Costa, M. & Furness, J.B. (1976) The peristaltic reflex: an analysis of the nerve pathways and their pharmacology. *Naunyn-Schmeidebergs Arch Pharmacol* **294**, 47–60.

Cottrell, D.F. & Iggo, A. (1984a) The response of duodenal tension receptors in sheep to pentagastrin, cholecystokinin and some other drugs. *J Physiol* **354**, 477–495.

Cottrell, D.F. & Iggo, A. (1984b) Mucosal enteroreceptors with vagal afferent fibres in the proximal duodenum of sheep. *J Physiol* **354**, 497–522.

Delbro, D., Fandriks, L., Rosell, S. & Folkers, K. (1983) Inhibition of antidromically induced stimulation of gastric motility by substance P receptor blockade. *Acta Physiol Scand* **118**, 309–316.

Delbro, D., Lissander, B. & Andersson, S.A. (1984) Atropine sensitive smooth muscle excitation by mucosal nociceptive stimulation—the involvement of an axon reflex? *Acta Physiol Scand* **122**, 621–627.

Dockray, G.J. & Sharkey, K.A. (1986) Neurochemistry of visceral afferent neurones. In Cervero, F. & Morrison, J.F.B. (eds), *Progress in Brain Research, Vol 67. Visceral Sensation*, pp. 133–148. Elsevier, Amsterdam.

Doerffler-Melly, J. & Neuhuber, W.L. (1988) Retrospinal neurons: evidence for a direct projection from the enteric to the central nervous system in the rat. *Neurosci Lett* **92**, 121–125.

Douglas, W.W. & Ritchie, J.M. (1957) On excitation of non-medullated afferent fibres in the vagus and aortic nerves by pharmacological agents. *J Physiol* **138**, 31–43.

Drapanas, T., McDonald, J.C. & Stewart, J.D. (1962) Serotonin release following instillation of hypertonic glucose into the proximal intestine. *Ann Surg* **156**, 528–536.

Dray, A., Bettaney, J., Forster, P. & Perkins, M.N. (1988) Bradykinin-induced stimulation of afferent fibres is mediated through protein kinase C. *Neurosci Lett* **91**, 301–307.

Durrans, S. & Taylor, T.V. (1986) The intragastric balloon, a new treatment for obesity. *Clin Nutr* **5**, 113–115.

Fandriks, L. & Delbro, D. (1983) Neuronal stimulation of gastric bicarbonate secretion in the cat. An involvement of vagal axon reflexes and substance P. *Acta Physiol Scand* **118**, 301–304.

Floyd, K., McMahon, S.B. & Morrison, J.F.B. (1982) Inhibitory interactions between colonic and vesical afferents in the micurition reflex in the cat. *J Physiol* **322**, 45–52.

Garattini, S., Mennini, T., Bendotti, G., Invernizzi, R. & Samanin, R. (1986) Neurochemical mechanisms of action of drugs which modify feeding via the serotonergic system. In Nicolaidis, S. (ed), *Serotonergic System, Feeding and Body Weight Regulation*, pp. 15–38. Academic Press, London.

German, V.F., Corrales, R., Veki, I.F. & Nadel, J.A. (1982) Reflex stimulation of tracheal mucus gland secretion by gastric irritation in cats. *J Appl Physiol* **52**, 1153–1155.

Gershon, M.D. & Erde, S.M. (1981) The nervous system of the gut. *Gastroenterology* **80**, 1571–1594.

Ginzel, K.H. (1973) Muscle relaxation by drugs which stimulate sensory nerve endings. The effect of veratrum alkaloids, phenyldiguanide and 5-hydroxytryptamine. *Neuropharmacol* **12**, 133–148.

Glaum, S.R., Proudfit, H.K. & Anderson, E.G. (1988) Reversal of the antinociceptive effects of intrathecally administered serotonin in the rat by a selective $5HT_3$ receptor antagonist. *Neurosci Lett* **95**, 313–317.

Govoni, S., Hanbauer, I., Hexum, T.D., Yang, T., Kelly, G.D. & Costa, E. (1981) *In vivo* characterization of the mechanisms that secrete enkephalin-like peptides stored in dog adrenal medulla. *Neuropharmacol* **20**, 639–645.

Gronstad, K.O., Ahlund, L., Dahlstrom, A., Haggendal, J. & Ahlman, H. (1988) A possible mechanism for the release of serotonin from the gut caused by pentagastrin. *J Surg Res* **44**, 473–478.

Grundy, D. (1988) Speculations on the structure/function relationship for vagal and splanchnic afferent endings supplying the gastrointestinal tract. *J Auton Nerv Syst* **22**, 175–180.

Grundy, D. & Davison, J.S. (1981) Cardiovascular changes elicited by vagal gastric afferents in the rat. *Q J Exp Physiol* **66**, 307–310.

Grundy, D. & Scratcherd, T. (1988) Sensory afferents from the gastrointestinal tract. In Wood, J.D. (ed), *Motility and Circulation of the Gastrointestinal Tract*. American Physiology Society, Bethesda MD.

Hardcastle, J.D. & Mann, C.V. (1968) Study of large bowel peristalsis. *Gut* **9**, 512–520.

Harper, A.A., Kidd, C., Scratcherd, T. (1959) Vagovagal reflex effects on gastric and pancreatic secretion and gastrointestinal motility. *J Physiol* **148**, 417–436.

Haupt, P., Jänig, W. & Kohler, W. (1983) Response pattern of visceral afferent fibres, supplying the colon, upon chemical and mechanical stimuli. *Pflügers Arch* **398**, 41–47.

Hawthorn, J., Andrews, P.L.R., Ang, V.T.Y. & Jenkins, J.S. (1988a) Differential release of vasopressin and oxytocin in response to abdominal vagal afferent stimulation or apomorphine in the ferret. *Brain Res* **438**, 193–198.

Hawthorn, J., Ostler, K.J. & Andrews, P.L.R. (1988b) The role of the abdominal visceral innervation and 5-hydroxytryptamine-M receptors in vomiting induced by the cytotoxic drugs cyclophosphamide and cisplatin in the ferret. *Q J Exp Physiol* **73**, 7–21.

Hewson, G., Leighton, G.E., Hill, R.G. & Hughes, J. (1988) The cholecystokinin receptor antagonist L364–718 increases food intake in the rat by attenuation of the action of endogenous cholecystokinin. *Br J Pharmacol* **93**, 79–84.

Higashi, H. (1986) Pharmacological aspects of visceral sensory receptors. In Cervero, F. & Morrison, J.F.B. (eds), *Progress in Brain Research, Vol 67. Visceral Sensation*, Elsevier, Amsterdam.

Holzer, P. & Sametz, W. (1986) Gastric mucosal protection against ulcerogenic factors in the rat mediated by capsaicin sensitive afferent neurons. *Gastroenterology* **91**, 975–981.

Jänig, W. & Morrison, J.F.B. (1986) Functional properties of spinal visceral afferents supplying abdominal and pelvic organs, with special emphasis on visceral nociception. Cervero, F. & Morrison, J.F.B. (eds), *Progress in Brain Research, Vol. 67. Visceral Sensation*, pp. 87–114. Elsevier, Amsterdam.

Jodal, M. & Lundgren, O. (1987) Effects of enterotoxins from *Vibrio cholerae* and *Escherichia coli* on intestinal motility and electrolyte transport. In Read, N.W. (ed), *The Relationships Between Intestinal Motility and Epithelial Transport*. Janssen Research Council, Beerse, Belgium.

Kaczmarek, L.K. (1987) The role of protein kinase C in the regulation of ion channels and neurotransmitter release. *Trends Neurosci* **10**, 30–34.

Kang, J.Y., Yap, I., Guan, R., Tay, H.H. & Math, M.V. (1989) Acid-induced duodenal ulcer pain: the influence of symptom status and the effect of an antispasmodic. *Gut* **30**, 166–170.

King, B.F. & Szurszewski, J.H. (1984) Mechanoreceptor pathways from the distal colon to the autonomic nervous system in the guinea-pig. *J Physiol* **350**, 93–107.

Kocher, L., Anton, F., Reeh, P.W. & Handwerker, H.O. (1987) The effects of carageenin-induced inflammation on the sensitivity of unmyelinated skin nociceptors in the rat. *Pain* **29**, 363–373.

Kukorelli, T. & Juhasz, G. (1976) Electroencephalographic synchronization induced by stimulation of small intestine and splanchnic nerve in cats. *Electroenceph Clin Neurophysiol* **44**, 491–500.

Kukorelli, T. & Juhasz, G. (1977) Sleep induced by intestine stimulation in cats. *Physiol Behav* **19**, 355–358.

Kumazawa, T. & Mizumura, K. (1984) Abnormal activity of polymodal receptors induced by clioquinol. *Brain Res* **310**, 185–188.

Kuo, D.C., Yang, G.C.H., Yamasaki, D.S. & Krauthamer, G.M. (1982) A wide field electron microscopic analysis of the fibre constituents of the major splanchnic nerve in the cat. *J Comp Neurol* **210**, 49–58.

Latimer, P., Campbell, D., Latimer, M., Sarna, S., Daniel, E. & Waterfall, W. (1979) Irritable bowel syndrome: a test of the colonic hyperalgesia hypothesis. *J Behav Med* **2**, 285–295.

Leape, L.L., Holder, T.M., Franklin, J.D., Amoury, R.A. & Ashcraft, K.W. (1977) Respiratory arrest in infants secondary to gastroesophageal reflux. *Paediatrics* **60**, 924–928.

Leslie, R.A. (1985) Neuroactive substances in the dorsal vagal complex of the medulla oblongata: nucleus of the tractus solitarius, area postrema and dorsal motor nucleus of the vagus. *Neurochem Int* **7**, 191–211.

Lew, W.Y.W. & Longhurst, J.C. (1986) Substance P, 5-hydroxytryptamine and bradykinin stimulate abdominal visceral afferents. *Am J Physiol* **250**, 465–473.

Lewis, T. (1942) *Pain*. Macmillan, London.

Lipkin, M. & Sleisenger, M.H. (1958) Studies of visceral pain: measurements of stimulus intensity and duration associated with the onset of pain in oesophagus, ileum and colon. *J. Clin Invest* 37, 28–34.

Llewellyn-Smith, I.J., Furness, J.B., Wilson, A.J. & Costa, M. (1983) Organization and fine structure of enteric ganglia. In Elvin, L.G. (ed), *Autonomic Ganglia*, pp. 145–182. Wiley, Chichester.

Longhurst, J.C., Ashton, J.H. & Iwamoto, G.A. (1980) Cardiovascular reflexes resulting from capsaicin stimulated gastric receptors in anaesthetized dogs. *Circ Res* 46, 780–788.

Longhurst, J.C., Spilker, H.L. & Ordway, G.A. (1981) Cardiovascular reflexes elicited by passive gastric distension in anaesthetized cats. *Am J Physiol* 240, 539–545.

Longhurst, J.C., Stebbins, C.L. & Ordway, G.A. (1984a) Chemically induced cardiovascular reflexes arising from the stomach in the cat. *Am J Physiol* 247, 459–466.

Longhurst, J.C., Kaufman, M.P., Ordway, G.A. & Musch, T.I. (1984b) Effect of bradykinin and capsaicin on endings of afferent fibres from abdominal visceral organs. *Am J Physiol* 247, 552–559.

Mackay, T.W. & Andrews, P.L.R. (1983) A comparative study of the vagal innervation of the stomach in man and the ferret. *J Anat* 136, 449–481.

Mei, N. (1985) Intestinal chemosensitivity. *Physiol Rev* 65, 211–237.

Mense, S. (1981) Sensitization of group IV muscle receptors to bradykinin by 5-hydroxytryptamine and prostaglandin E_2. *Brain Res* 225, 95–105.

Moss, H. & Sanger, G.J. (1987) Antagonism by BRL43694 of pseudoaffective reflexes evoked by duodenal distension. *Br J Pharmacol* 92, 531P.

Ness, T.J. & Gebhart, G.F. (1987) Characterization of neuronal responses to noxious visceral and somatic stimuli in the medial lumbosacral spinal cord of the rat. *J Neurophysiol* 57, 1867–1892.

Ness, T.J. & Gebhart, G.F. (1988a) Colorectal distension as a noxious visceral stimulus: physiologic and pharmacologic characterization of pseudoaffective reflexes in the rat. *Brain Res* 450, 153–169.

Ness, T.J. & Gebhart, G.F. (1988b) Characterization of neurons responsive to noxious colorectal distension in the spinal cord of the rat. *J Neurophysiol* 60, 1419–1438.

Neuhuber, W.L. (1987) Sensory vagal innervation of the rat oesophagus and cardia: a light and electron microscopic anterograde tracing study. *J Auton Nerv Syst* 20, 243–255.

Newson, B., Ahlman, H., Dahlstrom, A. & Nyhus, L.M. (1982) Ultrastructural observations in the rat ileal mucosa of possible epithelial 'taste cells' and submucosal sensory neurons. *Acta Physiol Scand* 114, 161–164.

Ohta, T., Nakazato, Y. & Ohga, A. (1985) Reflex control of gastric motility by the vagus and splanchnic nerves in the guinea-pig *in vivo*. *J Auton Nerv Syst* 14, 137–149.

Pack, R.J. & Widdicombe J.G. (1984) Amine containing cells of the lung. *Eur J Resp Dis* 65, 559–578.

Paintal, A.S. (1954) The response of gastric stretch receptors and certain other abdominal and thoracic vagal receptors to some drugs. *J Physiol* 126, 271–285.

Paintal, A.S. (1964) Effects of drugs on vertebrate mechanoreceptors. *Pharmacol Rev* 16, 341–380.

Pairet, M., Meirieu, O., Bardon, T. & Ruckebusch, Y. (1986) Cholinergic modulation of the release of serotonin in the gastric interstitial fluid: an *in vivo* study in rabbits. *Gastroenterology* 91, 1250–1257.

Pelchat, M.L. & Rozin, P. (1982) The special role of nausea in the acquisition of food dislikes by humans. *Appetite* 3, 341–351.

Petterson, G. (1979) The neural control of the serotonin content in mammalian enterochromaffin cells. *Acta Physiol Scand* (Suppl) 470, 1–30.

Resnick, R.H. & Gray, S.J. (1961) Distribution of serotonin in the human gastro-intestinal tract. *Gastroenterology* 41, 119–121.

Richter, J.E., Barish, C.F. & Castell, D.O. (1986) Abnormal sensory perception in patients with oesophageal chest pain. *Gastroenterology* 91, 845–852.

Ritchie, J. (1985) Mechanisms of pain in the irritable bowel syndrome. In Read, N.W. (ed), *Irritable Bowel Syndrome*, pp. 163–171. Grune & Stratton, London.

Rogers, J., Henry, M.M. & Nisiewicz, J.J. (1989) Increased segmented activity and intraluminal pressures in the sigmoid colon of patients with the irritable bowel syndrome. *Gut* 30, 634–641.

Russell, N.J.W., Schiable, H.G. & Schmidt, R.F. (1987) Opiates inhibit the discharges of fine afferent units from inflamed knee joint of the cat. *Neurosci Lett* 76, 107–112.

Sanger, G.J. & King, F.D. (1988) From metoclopramide to selective gut motility stimulants and 5HT$_3$ receptor antagonists. *Drug Des Delivery* 3, 273–295.

Sato, M. & Koyano, H. (1987) Autoradiographic study on the distribution of vagal afferent nerve fibres in the gastroduodenal wall of the rabbit. *Brain Res* 400, 101–109.

Schaible, H.G. & Schmidt, R.F. (1985) Effects of an experimental arthritis on the sensory properties of fine articular afferent units. *J Neurophysiol* 54, 1109–1122.

Schang, J.C., Dapoigny, M. & Devroede, G. (1987) Stimulation of colonic peristalsis by vasopressin: electromyographic study in normal subjects and patients with chronic idiopathic constipation. *Can J Physiol Pharmacol* 65, 2137–2141.

Sicuteri, F. (1968) Sensitization of nociceptors by 5-hydroxytryptamine in man. In Lim, R.K.S. (ed), *Proceedings of the 3rd International Congress of Pharmacology*, Pergamon Press, Oxford.

Sobue, I. (1979) Clinical aspects of subacute myelo-optic neuropathy (SMON). In Vinken, J. & Bruyn, G.W. (eds), *Handbook of Clinical Neurology, Vol. 37*, pp. 115–139. North Holland Publishing Co., Amsterdam.

Stern, R.M., Koch, K.L., Stewart, W.R. & Lindblad, I.M. (1987) Spectral analysis of tachygastria recorded during motion sickness. *Gastroenterology* 92, 92–97.

Thorbert, G., Alm, P. & Rosengren, E. (1978) Cyclic and steroid-induced changes in adrenergic neurotransmitter level of guinea-pig uterus. *Acta Obstet Gynaecol Scand* 57, 45–48.

Thorbert, G., Alm, P., Bjorklund, A., Owman, C. & Sjoberg, N.O. (1979) Adrenergic innervation of the human uterus. Disappearance of the transmitter and adrenergic transmitter forming enzymes during pregnancy. *Am J Obstet Gynaecol* 135, 223–226.

Ukai, M., Moran, W.H. & Zimmerman, B. (1968) The role of visceral afferent pathways on vasopressin secretion and urinary excretory patterns during surgical stress. *Ann Surg* 168, 16–28.

Watt, A.H., Lewis, D.J.M., Horne, J.J. & Smith, P.M. (1987) Reproduction of epigastric pain of duodenal ulceration by adenosine. *Br Med J* 294, 10–12.

Wiley, J., Tatum, D., Keinath, R. & Owyang, C. (1988) Participation of gastric mechanoreceptors and intestinal chemoreceptors in the gastrocolonic response. *Gastroenterology* 94, 1144–1149.

Wolf, S. (1965) *The Stomach*, p. 321. Oxford University Press, New York.

Wood, J.D. (1983) Neurophysiology of parasympathetic and enteric ganglia. In Elvin, L.G. (ed), *Autonomic Ganglia*. Wiley, Chichester.

11 *Hypnotic Desensitization of the Bowel*

P.J. Whorwell

Hypnosis is the subject of considerable controversy and there is not even a universally agreed definition of what it represents. There are 'state' and 'non-state' theorists, with the former firmly believing that it is some form of altered state of consciousness and the latter not taking such a rigid view (Naish, 1986). Unfortunately, until there is a test or physiological measurement that can confirm or refute its existence the arguments will continue. The situation is further confused by the protagonists of various allied techniques who insist that their method is unique in some way. It would seem much more likely that meditation, yoga, autogenic training, etc. are all variations on a similiar theme rather than being distinct entities. In addition it might be expected that a whole variety of induction techniques, both pleasant and even unpleasant, could result in the induction of the same 'state'. Thus it is possible that phenomena like mass hysteria may form part of the hypnotic spectrum. If the technique is going to be used for therapeutic gain it would seem logical to induce it in a pleasant way. Consequently, hypnotic induction methods usually employ attempts to concentrate the patient's mind on a single concept in combination with suggestions of comfort, relaxation and calm (Waxman, 1989). Our technique as applied to the gastrointestinal system has been described more fully elsewhere (Whorwell, 1991). It is important for all patients to realize that when hypnotized they are not unconscious in any way and are certainly not under the control of the hypnotherapist. I see hypnosis as a self-induced state for which the hypnotherapist is a catalyst. Indeed, the key to the therapeutic use of the technique is that the patient should rapidly learn the art of self-hypnosis.

The hypnosis literature is burdened down by extravagant claims and anecdotal reports on its efficacy in various conditions with hardly any controlled data. However, some observations suggest it has potential that is worthy of further exploration (Black *et al.*, 1963; Fry *et al.*, 1964; Maher-Loughnan, 1970, 1980; Deabler *et al.*, 1973; Clawson & Swade, 1975; Erickson, 1977; De Piano & Salzberg, 1979; Stacher *et al.*, 1980). The technique is only going to become more acceptable if it is subjected to scientific scrutiny and its role in modern medicine more clearly defined.

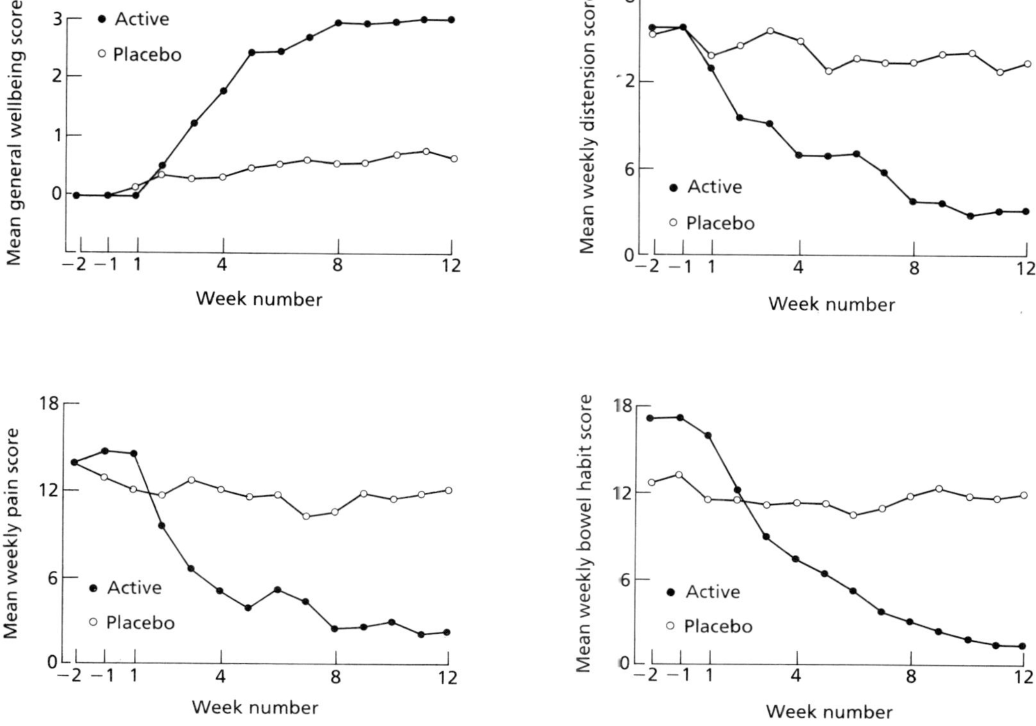

Fig. 11.1. Response of patients vs. controls to treatment with hypnotherapy. (Redrawn with permission from *The Lancet*.)

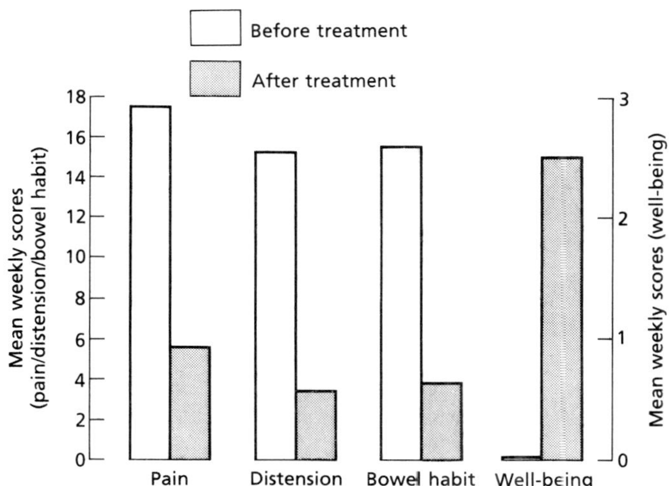

Fig. 11.2. Long-term follow-up of 50 patients treated with hypnotherapy. (Redrawn with permission from *Gut*.)

Table 11.1. Results for 50 patients treated with hypnotherapy

	Number	Improved	Not improved
Classic cases	38	36 (95%)	2
Atypical cases	7	3 (43%)	4
Classic cases with psychopathology	5	3 (60%)	2
Total	50	42 (84%)	8
Patients over age 50 from any group	8	2 (25%)	6

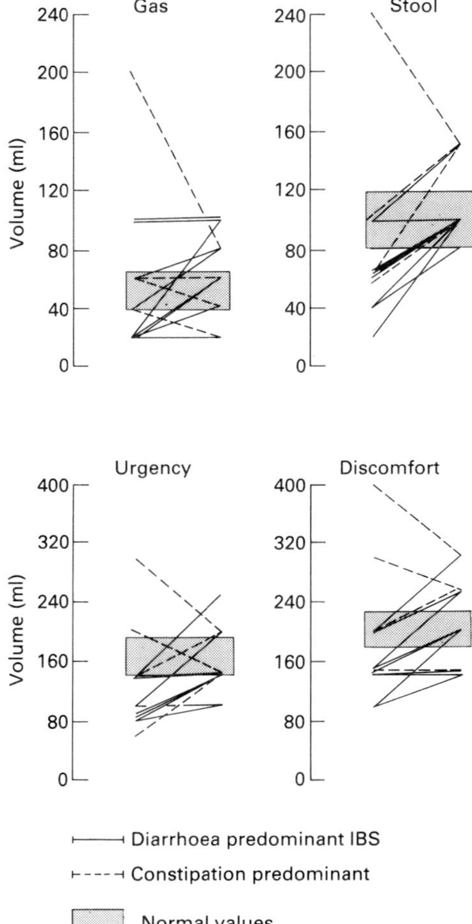

Fig. 11.3. Changes in rectal sensitivity following hypnotherapy.

In 1984 we reported the results of a clinical trial of the effect of hypnotherapy in patients with severe refractory irritable bowel syndrome (Whorwell *et al.*, 1984). Thirty patients who had failed to respond to conventional therapy were randomized to two groups, one of which received a course of hypnotherapy. After 3 months, compared with the controls the patients receiving hypnotherapy were much improved with respect to all the symptoms recorded (Fig. 11.1). Further long-term follow-up of the patients demonstrated that the beneficial effect was long-lasting (Whorwell *et al.*, 1987) although some patients appeared to need the occasional top-up session of hypnotherapy (Fig. 11.2). Response to treatment was difficult to predict, but patients in the older age groups, those with psychopathology and patients with atypical IBS seemed to do less well (Table 11.1). Recently Harvey *et al.* (1989) have independently confirmed our encouraging results and have also suggested that group therapy may be a practical proposition.

The mechanism by which hypnotherapy could be helping patients is speculative but is likely to be by a number of different mechanisms. For instance it probably reduces stress levels and increases coping ability. It is also possible that it might actually lead to some modification of gut responsiveness and we have recently reported a study that supports this view. Patients undergoing hypnotherapy for IBS were subjected to anorectal manometric assessment both before and after a course of therapy (Prior *et al.*, 1990a). Patients with visceral hypersensitivity (Prior *et al.*, 1990b) showed a significant reduction in this abnormality, whereas in those subjects with hyposensitivity there was a tendency to change in the opposite direction (Fig. 11.3).

As hypnotherapy is so time consuming it is at present only possible to offer treatment to subjects with severe refractory symptoms. However, this drawback may be overcome by the technique being made more widely available and by the use of group therapy. Investigation of the mechanism of action of hypnotherapy may not only increase its acceptability but also lead to new insights in the understanding of the pathophysiology of IBS.

REFERENCES

Black, S., Humphrey, J.H. & Niven, J.S.F. (1963) Inhibition of Mantoux reaction by direct suggestion under hypnosis. *Br Med J* 1, 1649–1651.

Clawson, T.A. & Swade, R.H. (1975) The hypnotic control of blood flow and pain. *Am J Clin Hypn* 17, 160–169.

De Piano, F.P. & Salzberg, H.C. (1979) Clinical applications of hypnosis in three psychosomatic disorders. *Psychol Bull* 86, 1223–1235.

Deabler, H.L., Fidel, E., Dillenkoffer, R.L. & Eider, S.T. (1973) The use of relaxation and hypnosis in lowering high blood pressure. *Am J Clin Hypn* 16, 75–83.

Erickson, M.H. (1977) Control of physiological functions by hypnosis. *Am J Clin Hypn* 20, 8–19.

Fry, L., Mason, A.A. & Pearson, R.S. (1964) Effect of hypnosis on allergic skin responses in asthma and hay fever. *Br Med J* 1, 1145–1148.

Harvey, R.F., Gunary, R.M., Hinton, R.A. & Barry, R.E. (1989) Individual and group hypnotherapy in the treatment of refractory IBS. *Lancet* 1, 424–425.

Maher-Loughnan, G.P. (1970) Hypnosis and autohypnosis for the treatment of asthma. *Int J Clin Exp Hypn* 12, 1–14.

Maher-Loughnan, G.P. (1980) Clinical applications of hypnosis in medicine. *Br J Hosp Med* 23, 447–455.

Naish, P.L.N. (1986) *What is Hypnosis—Current Theories and Research*. Open University Press, Milton Keynes.

Prior, A., Colgan, S.M. & Whorwell, P.J. (1990a) Changes in rectal sensitivity following hypnotherapy for irritable bowel syndrome. *Gut* 31, 896–898.

Prior, A., Maxton, D.G. & Whorwell, P.J. (1990b) Anorectal manometry in IBS: differences between diarrhoea- and constipation-predominant subjects. *Gut* 31, 458–462.

Stacher, G., Berner, P., Naske, R. *et al.* (1980) Effect of hypnotic suggestion of relaxation on basal and betazole-stimulated gastric acid secretion. *Dig Dis Sci* 25, 404–413.

Waxman, W. (ed), (1989) *Hartland's Medical and Dental Hypnosis*, 3rd edn. Baillière Tindall, London.

Whorwell, P.J. (1991) Hypnosis and the gastrointestinal system. *Brit J Hosp Med* 45, 27–29.

Whorwell, P.J., Prior, A. & Faragher, E.B. (1984) Controlled trial of hypnotherapy in the treatment of severe refractory irritable bowel syndrome. *Lancet* 2, 1232–1234.

Whorwell, P.J., Prior, A. & Colgan, S.M. (1987) Hypnotherapy of severe irritable bowel syndrome: further experience. *Gut* 28, 423–425.

Section 4
Immune Mechanisms and Food Intolerance

12 *The Immune System and the Irritable Gut*

J.R. Barton

Irritable bowel syndrome (IBS) is not a single disease entity, but a constellation of symptoms. As such it does not suggest any particular aetiology or pathology although there are several possible mechanisms. It may be the manifestation of a primary motility disorder, or the final common pathway for the expression of an abnormality of hormones, smooth muscle, psyche, or digestive enzymes. It may be secondary to a chemical or immune-mediated reaction to food, and some studies suggest that exclusion diets, often of multiple foods, may lead to improvement in up to 70% of patients with IBS. Possible roles and mechanisms of involvement of the immune system in the pathogenesis of IBS will be reviewed after a short description of normal gut mucosal immune physiology.

MUCOSAL AND SYSTEMIC IMMUNE RESPONSES TO ANTIGEN

The encounter between an antigen and the gastrointestinal immune system may lead to secretion of antibodies into the gut, cellular proliferation in the gut wall and a systemic response. The responses may be associated or independent. Current evidence suggests that the reaction to any particular antigen is regulated by a number of factors including (a) the nature of the antigen; (b) the dose of the antigen; (c) the copresentation of other antigens or adjuvants; (d) the timing and frequency of antigen encounter; and (e) the integrity of the gut itself.

How antigen reaches the immune apparatus will be discussed first, then the physiology and nature of the immune responses, followed by immune tolerance. Possible causes of disruption of gut mucosal physiology will be described with the subsequent immunopathology. Finally, immune abnormalities in gut diseases will be discussed, focusing on IBS and the role of dietary antigens.

Antigen uptake and sampling

It has long been recognized that immunoglobulins and other proteins fed to suckling animals can be found intact in serum

"

(Ganghofner & Langer, 1904); the gut of newborn infants in particular is more highly permeable (Beach *et al.*, 1982; Roberton *et al.*, 1982). Previously disputed to occur in adult humans (Amman & Stiehm, 1966; Kenny *et al.*, 1967; Krahenbuhl & Campiche, 1969), there is now evidence in favour of this; in fact continuous antigen uptake and sampling occurs, probably throughout the whole small bowel and to a lesser extent the large bowel (Iyengar & Selvaraj, 1972; Ogra *et al.*, 1977; Swarbrick *et al.*, 1979; Husby *et al.*, 1987).

Antigen is taken up mainly via specialized M cells (Dharakul *et al.*, 1988), which exist in the follicle-associated epithelium (FAE) that overlies lymphoid follicles (Owen *et al.*, 1986). The FAE has few goblet cells, a paucity of mucus and evidence of reduced local secretory antibody production (Pappo & Owen, 1988), all of which will facilitate antigen uptake. M cells have a poorly developed glycocalyx, thin apical cytoplasm and a central hollow in which a lymphocyte or macrophage may frequently be found. The M cells transport antigens from the gut lumen to the underlying lymphoid tissue in relatively intact form; the lack of phagolysosomes diminishes degradation of the transported antigens (Keljo & Hamilton, 1983). There is evidence that antigen may undergo subtle processing on its passage through the mucosa, a change which seems to render it more likely to induce tolerance, and which cannot be mimicked by systemic processing or *in vitro* physicochemical alteration (Bruce & Ferguson, 1986a, 1986b).

There may also be some leakage of molecules through the tight junctions between the enterocytes and this may increase dramatically in certain disease states, after ingestion of alcohol, and after non-steroidal anti-inflammatory drugs.

Antigen presentation

After crossing the gut mucosa, antigens gain access to the subepithelial space. There they are taken up by antigen presenting cells such as irregularly shaped, stellate, dendritic cells (Richman *et al.*, 1981) or macrophages, and processed for presentation to lymphocytes within the underlying Peyer's patch. Successful presentation depends upon the presence and copresentation of certain of the compatible class II major histocompatibility complex (MHC) antigens which are exhibited on the antigen presenting cells. The current view is that the antigen and the class II molecules are exhibited side by side on the surface of the antigen presenting cell and come into contact with receptors on the surface of the T cell. If the molecular configurations are compatible, an interaction occurs and the T cell is stimulated to respond. The class II antigens usually involved are of the DR group, and expression of these DR antigens on the antigen presenting cells can be induced by lymphokines, soluble protein messengers secreted by certain cells of the immune system (Wallach *et al.*, 1982); DR expression (and therefore perhaps increased antigen presentation) may also occur on enterocytes in certain disease states (Barclay & Mason, 1982; Pallone *et al.*, 1988); this may be part of their pathogenesis, or a bystander phenomenon.

The mechanism of the immune response

After T cells interact with the antigen presenting cells, they differentiate, and antigen-specific T cells then migrate from Peyer's patches to mesenteric lymph nodes (MLN) and, via the lymphoid tissue and thoracic duct, to the systemic circulation. These T cells may be of either helper or suppressor phenotype but what determines this is not known. From here they return to diffusely recolonize all mucosal tissues (salivary and tear glands, breast, bronchial and urogenital tissues, as well as the whole length of the gut) thus giving rise to the concept of a common mucosal immune system (MacDermott & Bienenstock, 1979). It has been shown that whilst widely migrating to mucosal lymphoid tissues there is preferential resettling in the tissue of origin (Guy-Grand *et al.*, 1978), mediated by specific interaction between molecules on the lymphocytes and specific receptors on the endothelium of high endothelial venules in the mucosal tissues (Kimpton *et al.*, 1989). These T cells then enter the lamina propria or epithelium. T helper cells are predominant in the lamina propria and T suppressor cells in the epithelium, i.e. intraepithelial lymphocytes (IELs) (Janossy *et al.*, 1980). These terminally differentiated antigen-specific cells are now *in situ* for appropriate help or suppression of the immune response by their influence over B cells following subsequent antigen encounter.

Undifferentiated B cells lie in the germinal centres of Peyer's patches prior to stimulation. Specific T helper cells probably stimulate these B cells to begin the maturation process, and a subtype of T helper cells called 'switch' cells may induce the B cells to change the class of immunoglobulin which they exhibit on their surface; this is known as isotype switching (Kawanishi *et al.*, 1983a). After this these post-switch Peyer's patch B cells probably then migrate to the MLNs and undergo terminal differentiation to become mature, immunoglobulin producing cells (Kawanishi *et al.*, 1983b). Stimulation with bacterial lipopolysaccharide (LPS), present as a sampled antigen within the mucosa, also seems to be an essential part of this differentiation process, and after this the cells may then go on to repopulate the lamina propria and other components of the mucosal associated lymphoid tissue in the same fashion as the circulating T cells. Thus mucosal tissues become populated by both mature T and B antigen-specific lymphocytes differentiated and primed to respond to antigen challenge (Allansmith *et al.*, 1983;

Cruz & Hanson, 1983). Most antigens encountered are not harmful, e.g. food protein antigens and therefore the immune response must vary with respect to each particular antigen. A system of control exists to ensure this and, although the exact mechanisms of this control are unclear, regulation through a balance of T helper and T suppressor activity is implicated.

The immune response—what actually happens?

Most commonly after oral ingestion of antigen, specific antibodies may be detected in secretions (Challacombe & Tomasi, 1980). Antibodies of the IgA isotype predominate although some IgG and IgM antibodies are produced. Usually little or no serum antibody response is seen (Clancy *et al.*, 1983; Smith & Taubman, 1987).

There are a number of modulating influences on the physiology of this antigen encounter. The primary route of antigen encounter is important, with oral or intraintestinal immunization producing a secretory antibody response, and parenteral immunization little or no secretory response at all (Baumann *et al.*, 1985; Kurz *et al.*, 1986; Smith *et al.*, 1986; Waldman *et al.*, 1986). For a substantial secretory IgA response at least one enteric antigen encounter is necessary (Pierce, 1978). IgG secretory antibody responses may result when antigen is given by injection into Peyer's patches, the IgA antibody only appearing after a further stimulation by a second immunization. This suggests that the gut wall itself must be traversed to stimulate a primary IgA response (Dahlgren, 1987). A systemic immune response may also be seen after enteric antigen encounter (Rothberg *et al.*, 1973), with the primary encounter resulting in IgA antibodies rather than those of the IgG or IgM class. Although systemic IgA antibodies may occur, the nature of the IgA molecule does not incite an inflammatory reaction (Bazin *et al.*, 1970). In addition to exciting a humoral response, enteric immunization may also prime cytotoxic T cell precursors in the systemic immune system (Kagnoff, 1978a). If the original priming was parenteral, then the predominant systemic response is of the IgG isotype with the potential accompanying inflammatory reaction.

The specific secretory antibody response may increase with further antigen challenge, and can be dose-dependent (Carlsson *et al.*, 1985, Gregory & Filler, 1987). However, even a single oral immunization may lead to significant specific secretory antibody levels to certain antigens, e.g. dietary lectins (Gibbons & Dankers, 1986). Conversely, little or no antibody response may be invoked by other antigens such as soluble food proteins. Although secretory priming may occur after one or two exposures to antigen, repeated mucosal exposure may eventually lead to down-regulation of the secretory IgA response (Holt *et al.*, 1987). Concurrent administration of

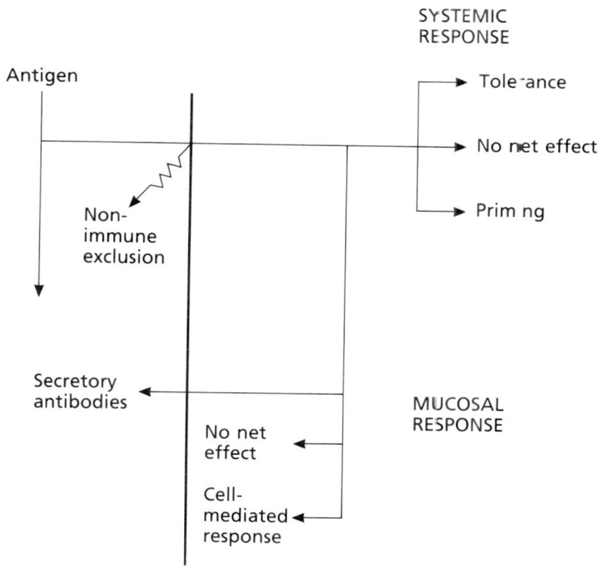

Fig. 12.1. Possible responses to gut-encountered antigens.

other substances such as adjuvants may influence the secretory
response. Coadministration of muramyl dipeptide for example
enhances the salivary specific antibody reponse to *Streptococcus
mutans*. Similarly, incomplete Freund's adjuvant enhances the
response to ovalbumin (Taubman *et al.*, 1983) and aluminium
phosphate to *S. mutans* glucosyltransferase (Smith & Taubman,
1987). Keyhole limpet haemocyanin, cholera and bacterial LPS may
all alter the immune response (McGhee *et al.*, 1982), perhaps by
facilitating T suppressor cell activation. Manoeuvres which may
prolong antigen life and therefore exposure to the gut immune
apparatus (such as incorporation into liposomes, which seems to
provide a 'slow-release' preparation) incite an enhanced specific
secretory IgA immune response (Wachsman *et al.*, 1985). The
possible responses are summarized in Fig. 12.1.

The mechanism of tolerance

Initial antigen encounter by the enteric route will frequently lead to
a decreased humoral and cellular response when that antigen is
subsequently presented systemically (Kagnoff, 1978b, 1978c, 1981,
1982). After oral antigen priming, specific T suppressor cells are
found in Peyer's patches, MLNs and, after prolonged exposure, in
the spleen (Mattingly & Waksman, 1978). It seems that hypo-
responsiveness may be mediated by either these T suppressor cells
or by antigen–antibody complexes or circulating antibodies. After
dietary protein feeding, tolerance seems mainly to be mediated by

T suppressor cells (Ngan & Kind, 1978), whereas after red cell antigen feeding, antibody–antigen complexes and circulating antibodies are also thought to be responsible (Andre *et al.*, 1974; Kagnoff, 1978c).

Systemic tolerance coupled to a secretory reaction with the production of specific intestinal IgA antibodies may be the most common response (Challacombe & Tomasi, 1980). However, recent work suggests independent regulation (Barton *et al.*, 1989a).

Antigen sorting

Just how the gut mucosal immune system distinguishes between antigens is not known. It may depend on the initial site of the antigen encounter with disruption of mucosal integrity leading to primary stimulation of the lamina propria or IELs instead of Peyer's patches. The dose of the antigen may be important (Lamont *et al.*, 1989) as may its nature. Monosaccharides, amino acids and oligopeptides, end products of normal digestion and the usual forms in which food is eventually absorbed across the gut wall, are of low antigenic potential. Incomplete digestion leaves polysaccharides, polypeptides or wholly unchanged foodstuffs which appear to be more highly antigenic (the optimum size for antigenicity for protein is about 5–6 amino acids long). Disruption of normal digestion, or increased permeability secondary to an insult, may therefore increase the access of these more antigenic molecules to the gut immune tissue (Ferguson & Carswell, 1972).

IMMUNE DISRUPTION OF THE GUT

Mechanisms

Any number of insults of a variety of types may potentially lead to disruption of normal antigen handling. Several non-specific mechanisms exist to inactivate and degrade gut antigens for protection against pathogens (Udall & Allan Walker, 1987) (see Table 12.1). These mechanisms usually ensure that antigen which reaches the mucosa is not live or toxic, and is generally of a sufficiently small molecular size as to be of low antigenicity. Disruption of any of the components of this system leads to increased access to the mucosa, not only to the agent of insult itself but also to other unrelated antigens, derived, for example, from foods or commensal bacteria. Bypass of the usual route of access may lead to abnormalities of immunoregulation and the failure of development of tolerance (Table 12.2). The mucosa becomes primed with antigenspecific T cells, B cells, plasma cells and mast cells. Secretory antibodies and cellular responses in the mucosa, in addition to serum antibody formation, may result. A primary parenteral en-

Table 12.1. Non-immune gastrointestinal protection

Gastric acid
Proteases
  Pancreatic
  Intestinal
Motility
Mucus layer
Enterocyte shedding and renewal
Intact enterocyte sheet

Table 12.2. Possible mechanisms and causes of immune disruption of the gut

Situation	Mechanism		Cause
Enterocyte damage		Antigen stimulation via permeability or access	Infection; bacterial overgrowth; ischaemia; drugs; malnutrition; IBD; coeliac disease
Increased/ abnormal antigenic stimulation	1	Incomplete food protein digestion	As above, plus: enzyme deficiencies with LPS; toxins; adjuvants
	2	Copresentation	
	3	Enterocyte HLA-DR expression and antigen presentation	Cytokines
	4	Failure of normal tolerance	Bypass of gut wall permeability; T_s cell abnormalities

IBD = inflammatory bowel disease. LPS = bacterial lipopolysaccharide.

counter with antigen might also prime the mucosa, and lead to the appearance of antigen-specific T cells in the gut, since the segregation of the mucosal and systemic immune compartments seems to occur only when antigen is first encountered via the gut and not when that encounter is parenteral. The mechanisms of this priming rather than the usual down-regulation are not known, but speculatively may be due to failure of activation of T suppressor cells, or copresentation of other antigens accessing the mucosa acting as adjuvants.

The role of IgA

The most important immunoglobulin in the mucosa, IgA, is also designed to diminish any inflammatory reactions which ensue. Functionally, secretory IgA in the intestinal lumen binds to and prevents bacterial adherence to enterocytes and thereby mucosal penetration. The secretory IgA appears to protect against viral infection and colonization (Ogra & Karzon, 1969). Lastly, it can reduce the passage of protein antigens across the mucosa (Andre *et al.*, 1974). Since IgA does not fix complement or have opsonizing activity, it neither effectively kills cells nor excites an inflammatory response. It is relatively ineffective at mediating antibody dependent cell-mediated cytotoxicity (Kagnoff & Campbell, 1976). This seems to link with the overall scheme of the down-regulation of immune response at mucosal level, IgA antibodies acting largely perhaps by exclusion and complexing rather than in stimulating an immune reaction.

In secretory IgA deficiency enhanced mucosal penetration by dietary antigens leads to increased circulating immune complexes and high serum anti-food protein antibody titres (Cunningham-Rundles *et al.*, 1979). This may be pathophysiological: there is an increased occurrence of atopic disorders in individuals with IgA deficiency, and their severity may be increased (Taylor *et al.*, 1973). There is also an association with a number of other disorders, e.g. allergic disorders, autoimmune diseases, connective tissue diseases and malignancy. Secretory IgA deficiency may be permanent or transient, and genetic or acquired, with certain drugs and even cigarette smoking having profound effects (Barton *et al.*, 1989b).

Hypersensitivity reactions in the gut

When normal defensive mechanisms have been breached and the gut is therefore primed, tissue damage may result from subsequent antigen exposure. The gut becomes the area of tissue damage although the site of entry of the antigen may be either enteral or parenteral. Two main types of hypersensitivity account for many of the important reactions occurring in the gut mucosa, immediate (type I) and delayed (type IV).

Immediate hypersensitivity

This type I hypersensitivity reaction may need only small amounts of antigen to trigger the response. The reaction is mediated via antigen binding to several specific surface IgE antibodies on the mast cell, leading to cross-linking of the IgE and subsequent degranulation of the mast cell. Current thinking suggests that there may be two phases to this response, instant and delayed, and although the late phase is probably not due to IgE it is convenient to mention it here. After IgE cross-linking, preformed mediators are released and excite an instant response, but other mediators may need to be synthesized and therefore are released more slowly over a few hours.

This late phase response creates diagnostic problems since, as it is impossible to predict the time interval from exposure to a food to the onset of symptoms, it is also difficult to implicate any one food as the culprit. Delayed or late phase hypersensitivity may be mediated by IgE, but is usually not (Middleton *et al.*, 1983), and therefore the current tests in use will not identify such a reaction (Ford, 1983). IgM, IgA and IgG (particularly subclass 4) are thought to be the relevant antibody isotypes (Middleton *et al.*, 1983). Specific IgG_4 antibody to allergen is raised in patients with food allergy, and is also high in patients diagnosed as allergic who have normal IgE levels and negative skin-prick and IgE-RAST tests (Halpern & Scott, 1987; Molkou & Waguet, 1981). IgG_4 receptors are found on basophils and mast cells (Nakagawa & deWeck, 1983). Other studies have implicated complement activation by IgG-immune complexes (Chang *et al.*, 1981). Good evidence from recent studies suggests that the late phase response may be due to a T cell dependent reaction (A.B. Kay, personal communication). A combination of the above factors is possible.

Whatever the trigger, mediator release induces increases in mucosal and capillary permeability. An inflammatory cascade then occurs with a magnified non-specific response resulting from the initial antigen-specific event. The gut itself becomes oedematous and epithelial damage can take place. Dramatic changes in sodium, chloride, potassium and water flux can occur, and plasma also leaks from the gut into the lumen (Russell & Castro, 1985). There is leakage of food proteins into the mucosa (Roberts *et al.*, 1981). These changes may lead to the symptoms in some cases of food allergy.

Delayed type hypersensitivity

On antigen encounter in a sensitized gut, there is an influx of T cells into the lamina propria and epithelium. An increase in crypt cell production rate occurs, and enterocyte transport up the villi accelerates. If the reaction is severe, crypt hyperplasia and villus shortening may take place. Disaccharidase deficiency is often seen in conjunction with these changes, reflecting enterocyte immaturity. An increased proportion of enterocytes are shown to express HLA-DR antigens on their surface, induced by γ-interferon released by antigen-stimulated T cells. Clinical examples of this cell-mediated reaction are coeliac disease and graft vs. host disease.

THE RELEVANCE TO GUT DISEASE

Introduction

The immune pathology in a selected sample of gut diseases which are at least in part immune-mediated is discussed below for the purpose of illuminating potential mechanisms of disruption of

Table 12.3. Examples of reactions to foods (see standard text, Brostoff &
Challacombe, (1987), for comprehensive details)

Psychological
Food avoidance/aversion

Intolerance
Pharmacological
    Caffeine (coffee, tea, carbonated drinks)
    Monosodium glutamate (Chinese food)
    Tyramine (cheese, wine)
    Salicylates
    Histamine (strawberries, shellfish)
Enzyme defect
    Lactase deficiency
    G6PD deficiency

Immune (allergy)
Immediate
    Mast cell degranulation (local and systemic effects)
    Late phase? IgG_4
Delayed, cell-mediated

the normal physiology. Cow's milk protein and soy protein enter-
opathies or colitis will not be covered, nor will eosinophilic gastroenteritis. The discussion will be confined to food allergy in general,
coeliac disease and IBS.

Food allergy

True food allergy in the immunological sense of the term is rare.
We would do well to remember and employ the definitions and
terminology of food-related reactions suggested by a recent joint
report (Royal College of Physicians, 1984). Food-related reactions
are classified into three categories:

1 Psychological food avoidance, where a patient experiences an
unpleasant reaction to a food which does not occur on blind testing, and which can be reproduced by administering a placebo but
suggesting to the patient that it is the food in question.

2 Food intolerance, where there is an unpleasant reproducible
response to blinded food challenge based on a chemical reaction.

3 True food allergy, where an adverse, reproducible, immunologically mediated response to food is demonstrated (see Table 12.3
for examples of these reactions).

If immune mechanisms are involved, how might that be? If the
normal physiology of the intestine is disturbed via mechanisms
discussed above, an immune reaction to antigenic foods might and
sometimes does occur and has been shown in some instances to lead
to histological change. Shortening and broadening of villi, crypt
hyperplasia, an indistinct brush border, and increased IEL numbers
have been observed (Shiner *et al.*, 1975; Iyngkaran *et al.*, 1978).

Occasionally, degenerative cells with vacuolated cytoplasm can be seen, and oedema and infiltration in the lamina propria has been noted with increased numbers of plasma cells, lymphocytes and mucosal mast cells. Mucosal mast cells are degranulated in increased numbers and plasma cells have dilated cisternae suggesting increased immunoglobulin production. Reports exist of high IgE cell numbers found in the mucosa after antigen challenge and of high IgA and IgM levels (Shiner *et al.*, 1975; Harris *et al.*, 1977; Burgin-Wolff *et al.*, 1980). There is no evidence of an increase in IgG in the tissues, however, a more likely candidate in terms of tissue destruction.

On the biochemical level these changes may lead to decreased disaccharidase activity. Recovery of the histological and biochemical abnormalities is very variable and depends on a number of factors such as age, persistence of infection and the presence of malnutrition. In infants recovery may take from 6 weeks to 6 months. Recovery may occur despite continued ingestion of the antigenic food proteins which were implicated in the initial pathophysiology, and paradoxically it may even occur more rapidly when these antigenic foods are ingested than when they are not. Often more than one food protein is implicated but, despite the example above, there is usually prompt response to withdrawal of the offending food proteins. Foods most frequently implicated in allergic reactions are milk, eggs, nuts and seafood. Full details have recently been reviewed by Iyngkaran & Yadav (1987).

There may be a macroscopic reaction observable, as in one endoscopic study where the offending allergens were applied to the gastric mucosa. Mucosal swelling, erosions and bleeding occurred, mast cell counts and histamine concentrations fell from high levels, and a lymphocyte infiltrate was seen (Reimann & Lewin, 1988).

The reactions may not be confined to the gut wall and extra-intestinal manifestations may be present. Further complicating factors are that some patients develop similar (milder) histological and biochemical changes and yet do not have any symptoms. The amounts of antigen required to precipitate these reactions seem to be unimportant; very small amounts have been shown to do so. The diagnosis of food allergy therefore remains a lengthy clinical process, preferably via an elemental diet followed by gradual reintroduction of foods one by one, or best of all by giving powdered foods in capsules in a double-blind manner. However, food allergy is much less common after the first few years of life, and is rarely proven in adults at present given the difficulties described.

Coeliac disease

Of all food allergies, coeliac disease is by far the best studied. Within a very short time of mucosal encounter of gluten, immune-mediated changes are apparent. An inflammatory infiltrate begins in the lamina propria and epithelium, consisting of T cells, eosinophils, basophils and mast cells. Crypt hyperplasia follows, with villus shortening and ultimately flattening. Serum antibodies to gliadin and other foods are high, as are secretory antibodies (Barton & Ferguson, 1988; O'Mahony *et al.*, 1990a). There is an increase in permeability of both the gut wall and the microvasculature, and a firm association with IgA deficiency which occurs in up to one in 40 patients (Asquith *et al.*, 1969).

Withdrawal of gluten leads to healing of the lesion, with decrease of serum antibody levels, although secretory antibodies may remain high for prolonged periods (O'Mahony *et al.*, 1989). Histological changes revert, some extremely slowly over 12 or more months, but subtle abnormalities may remain, with persistently raised IEL counts. The high secretory antibodies and IEL counts may be markers of persistent exposure to minute amounts of gluten, an expression of prolonged mucosal immunological memory, or part of the primary abnormality. High antibody titres to other food protein antigens are seen, however, and the histological abnormalities are not specific to coeliac disease. Any underlying defect in immunoregulation which leads on to gluten sensitivity remains undetected.

Irritable bowel syndrome

It is conceivable that some patients with IBS may derive a contribution to their disturbance in bowel habit from an immune-mediated reaction to food. The evidence implicating food is conflicting, some groups suggesting that allergy to foods leads to symptoms in as many as 70% of patients (Hunter *et al.*, 1985), perhaps especially in atopic subjects (Petit-Pierre *et al.*, 1985), whilst others believe it to be less important (Bentley *et al.*, 1983; Farah *et al.*, 1985) particularly in those patients with constipation (McKee *et al.*, 1987).

In a large study (Nanda *et al.*, 1989), 189 patients with refractory IBS were asked to exclude rigidly certain foods. Ninety-one patients' (48%) symptoms improved on the exclusion diet at 3 weeks, and of 73 still adhering to the diet at a mean 14.7 months, 72 were still improved. Of the 98 non-responders, 95 remained symptomatic. It is not clear if the non-responders were seen as frequently by a dietician and doctor as the responders during follow-up, and assessment of symptoms would have been better by visual analogue scale rather than by a four point questionnaire; however, this remains a significant study, suggesting that reaction to food is important in IBS. Unfortunately, no biochemical or immune parameters were studied.

Disruption of normal physiology may certainly result in immune reactions in the gut, and some food proteins are known to be pathological (e.g. gluten, soy, cow's milk protein) giving rise to reactions which may manifest themselves as abdominal pain or diarrhoea, etc. Investigation is difficult, hindered by the lack of any good diagnostic serum marker or test. Of the two widely used tests, skin-prick tests have proved to be unreliable (Lehmann, 1980), and IgE-RAST testing only has a sensitivity of between 12% and 50%. Standardization of the antigen extracts is difficult. A further problem is that many reactions to foods may well be caused by a late phase reaction, which occurs after a variable period and for which there is no marker.

The four studies which have addressed the inter-relationship between food and IBS give variable results. Patients with a diagnosis of IBS were put on an open exclusion diet followed by food challenge. Consistent responders were then forwarded to blinded challenge. In the earliest study, 25 patients entered, 21 completing the exclusion diet, 14 benefiting from it symptomatically. Six were randomized to blind challenge, confirming a reaction. However, no change in immune parameters was recorded in terms of serum eosinophil count, histamine level, IgE level and immune complexes. The rises in stool wet weight and rectal prostaglandin E_2 in fact suggest a non-immunological mechanism (Jones *et al.*, 1982). The second study of 27 patients confirmed food allergy in three, all of whom had presented initially with atopic symptoms (Bentley *et al.*, 1983). The third study of 24 patients (12 atopic) found 14 with symptoms reproducible on blind testing; of these, nine patients (who were all atopic) had evidence of an allergic mechanism with high IgE levels or a positive skin test (Petit-Pierre *et al.*, 1985). The most recent study of 10 patients found not one who responded to blinded challenge, despite six with positive skin tests (Zwetchkenbaum & Burakoff, 1988).

Further evidence against a significant immunological role for food in IBS comes from other studies, where immunoglobulin levels are normal in patients with IBS and diarrhoea (whereas they are raised in atopic patients with food intolerance, for example) and finally intestinal biopsies have revealed no differences (Lessof *et al.*, 1980). There are unexplored areas and, although some studies have used patients with IBS as controls for patients with coeliac disease when counting mast cells (Strobel *et al.*, 1983), the role of mast cells in IBS has not been specifically addressed.

SUMMARY

Thus it can be imagined how the immune response may be influenced by infection, ischaemia, malnutrition and drugs amongst other insults, with a subsequent inappropriate immune reaction. Disease states such as dietary protein intolerance, coeliac disease, cow's milk protein enteropathy, inflammatory bowel disease or even systemic allergic reactions may result. It is difficult to ascertain if the high food antibody titres frequently seen in these conditions are primary or secondary. Further mechanisms can be envisaged in which the normal tolerance to encountered oral antigens is disrupted; an inherited or aquired IgA deficiency, diminished mucosal defenses, deficiency of mucus, alteration in T cell function, impaired digestion and breakdown of food, or any state which induces a temporary or permanent inflammatory response in the intestine may do so. Changes in gut motor or secretory function as a result of immune reactions may occur, but there is no evidence of these alterations in IBS at present.

The picture is at present incomplete, and a pathophysiological role for immune activation in the gastrointestinal tract cannot be excluded as an aetiological mechanism in IBS. The presently available studies may not have investigated the relevant parameter at the relevant time, methodolgies used are crude, intestinal biopsies are not of the mid- or distal small bowel where major pathological alterations might occur, and the secretory side of the immune response has been almost totally neglected because of problems of access, ethics, and techniques. Hopefully newer methodologies, which are becoming available, will fill in these gaps (Barton *et al.*, 1990a; O'Mahony *et al.*, 1990b).

REFERENCES

Allansmith, M.R., Ebersole, J.L. & Burns, C.A. (1983) IgA antibody levels in human tears, saliva, and serum. *Ann N Y Acad Sci* **409**, 766–768.

Amman, A.J. & Stiehm, E.R. (1966) Immune globulin levels in colostrum and breast milk, and serum from formula- and breast-fed newborns. *Proc Soc Exp Biol Med* **122**, 1098–1100.

Andre, C., Andre, F., Bazin, H. & Heremans, J.F. (1974) Interference of oral immunization with the intestinal absorbtion of heterologous albumin. *Eur J Immunol* **4**, 701–704.

Asquith, P., Thompson, R.A. & Cooke, W.T. (1969) Serum immunoglobulins in adult coeliac disease. *Lancet* **ii**, 129–131.

Barclay, N.A. & Mason, D.W. (1982) Induction of IgA antigen in rat epidermal cells and gut epithelium by immunological stimuli. *J Exp Med* **156**, 1665–1676.

Barton, J.R. & Ferguson, A. (1988) Do salivary antibodies to dietary antigens reflect inappropriate stimulation of GALT or hyperpermeability?. In MacDermott, R.P. (ed), *Inflammatory Bowel Disease: Current Status and Future Approach*, pp. 213–217. Elsevier, Amsterdam.

Barton, J.R., O'Mahony, S. & Ferguson, A. (1990) Regulation of antibodies to food proteins within the common mucosal immune system: lack of correlation between antibody titres in saliva and intestinal fluid. In MacDonald, T.T., Challacombe, S.J., Bland, P.W., Stokes, C.R., Heatley, R.V. & Mowat A.McI., (eds), *Advances in Mucosal Immunology*, pp. 495–496. Kluwer Academic Publishers, Lancaster.

Barton, J.R., Riad, M.A., Gaze, M.N., Maran, A.G.D. & Ferguson, A. (1990b) Mucosal immunodeficiency in smokers and in patients with epithelial head and neck tumours. *Gut* **31**, 378–392.

Baumann, E., Binder, B.R., Falk, W., Huber, E.G., Kurz, R. & Rosanelli, K. (1985) Development and clinical use of an oral heat-inactivated whole cell pertussis vaccine. *Dev Biol Stand* **61**, 511–516.

Bazin, H., Levi, G. & Doria, G. (1970) Predominant contribution of IgA-antibody-forming cells to an immune response detected in extraintestinal tissues of germ free mice exposed to antigen by the oral route. *J Immunol* **105**, 1049–1051.

Beach, R.C., Menzies I.S., Clayden, G.S. & Scopes, J.W. (1982) Gastrointestinal permeability changes in the preterm neonate. *Arch Dis Child* **57**, 141–145.

Bentley, S.J., Pearson, D.J. & Rix, K.J.B. (1983) Food hypersensitivity in IBS. *Lancet* **ii**, 295–296.

Brostoff, J. & Challacombe, S. (1987) (eds), *Food Allergy and Intolerance*. Baillière Tindall, London.

Bruce, M & Ferguson, A. (1986a) Oral tolerance to ovalbumin in mice: studies of chemically modified and 'biologically filtered' antigen. *Immunology* **57**, 627–630.

Bruce, M.G. & Ferguson, A. (1986b) The influence of intestinal processing on the immunogenicity and molecular size of absorbed, circulating ovalbumin in mice. *Immunology* **59**, 295–300.

Burgin-Wolff, A., Sigver, E., Freiss, H., *et al.* (1980) The diagnostic significance of antibodies to various cow's milk proteins. *Eur J Pediatr* **133**, 17–24.

Carlson, J.R., Heyworth, M.F. & Owen, R.L. (1985) Relationship between Peyer's patch T cells and clearance of *Giardia* infection. *Gastroenterology* **88**, 1343 (abstract).

Challacombe, S.J. & Tomasi, T.B. (1980) Systemic tolerance and secretory immunity after oral immunization. *J Exp Med* **152**, 1459–1472.

Chang, T.T., Char, D.H. & Frick, O.L. (1981) Immune complexes in delayed onset food allergy. *J Allergy Clin Immunol* **67**, 4 (abstract).

Clancy, R.L., Cripps, A.W., Husband, A.J. & Buckley D. (1983) Specific immune response in the respiratory tract after administration of an oral polyvalent bacterial vaccine. *Infect Immun* **39**, 491–496.

Cruz, J.R. & Hanson, L.A. (1983) Specific immune response in human milk to oral immunization with food proteins. *Ann NY Acad Sci* **409**, 808–809.

Cunningham-Rundles, C., Brandeis, W.E., Good, R.A. & Day N.K. (1979) Bovine antigens and the formation of circulating immune complexes in selective IgA deficiency. *J Clin Invest* **64**, 272–279.

Dahlgren, U.I.H. (1987) Induction of salivary antibody response in rats after immunization in Peyer's patches. *Scand J Immunol* **26**, 193–96.

Dharakul, T., Riepenhoff-Talty, M., Albini, B. & Ogra, P.L. (1988) Distribution of rotavirus antigen in the intestinal lymphoid tissues: potential role in development of the mucosal immune response to rotavirus. *Clin Exp Immunol* **74**, 14–19.

Farah, D.A., Calder, I., Benson, L. & Mackenzie, J.F. (1985) Specific food intolerance: its place as a cause of gastrointestinal symptoms. *Gut* **26**, 164–168.

Ferguson, A. & Carswell, F. (1972) Precipitins to dietary proteins in serum and upper intestinal secretions in coeliac children. *Br Med J* **1**, 75–79.

Ford, R.P.K. (1983) Cow's milk hypersensitivity: immediate and delayed onset clinical patterns. *Arch Dis Child* **58**, 856–862.

Ganghofner, V. & Langer, J. (1904) Ueber die Resorption genuiner Eineisskorper im Magendarmkanal neugeborener Tiere und Säuglinge. *Munch Med Wochenschr* **34**, 1497–1502.

Gibbons, R.J. & Dankers, I. (1986) Immunosorbent assay of interactions between human parotid immunoglobulin A and dietary lectins. *Arch Oral Biol* **31**, 477–81.

Gregory, R.L. & Filler, S.J. (1987) Protective secretory immunoglobulin A antibodies in humans following oral immunization with *Streptococcus mutans*. *Infect Immun* **55**, 2409–15.

Guy-Grand, D., Griscelli, C. & Vassalli, P. (1978) The mouse gut T lymphocyte, a novel type of T cell. Nature, origin, and traffic *J Exp Med* **148**, 1661–1667.

Halpern, G.M. & Scott, J.R. (1987) Non-IgE antibody mediated mechanisms in food allergy. *Ann Allergy* **58**, 14–27.

Harris, M.J., Petts, B. & Penny, R. (1977) Cow's milk allergy as a cause of infantile colic: immunofluorescence study on jejunal mucosa. *Aust Pediatr J* 13, 276–281.

Holt, P.G., Reid, M., Britten, D., Sedgwick, J. & Bazin, H. (1987) Suppression of IgE responses by passive antigen inhalation: dissociation of local (mucosal) and systemic immunity. *Cell Immunol* 104, 434–39.

Hunter, J.O., Workman, E. & Alun Jones, V. (1985) Dietary studies. In Gibson, P.R. & Jewell, D.P. (eds), *Topics in Gastroenterology 12*, pp. 305–315. Blackwell Scientific Publications, Oxford.

Husby, S., Svehag, S-E. & Jensenius, J.C. (1987) Passage of dietary antigens in man: kinetics of appearance in serum and characterization of free and antibody-bound antigen. *Adv Exp Med Biol* 216A, 801–812.

Iyengar, L. & Selvaraj, R.J. (1972) Intestinal absorption of immunoglobulins by newborn infants. *Arch Dis Child* 47, 411–414.

Iyngkaran, N. & Yadav, M. (1987) Food allergy. In Marsh, M.N. (ed), *Immunopathology of the Small Intestine*, pp. 415–449. Wiley, Chichester.

Iyngkaran, N., Robinson, M.J., Sumithran, E., Lam, S.K., Puthucheary, S.D. & Yadav, M. (1978) Cow's milk protein sensitive enteropathy: an important factor in prolonging diarrhoea of acute infective enteritis in early infancy. *Arch Dis Child* 53, 150–153.

Janossy, G., Tidman, N., Selby, W.S. *et al.* (1980) Human T lymphocytes of inducer and suppressor type occupy different microenvironments. *Nature* 288, 81–844.

Jones, A.V., Shorthouse, M., McLaughan, P. *et al.* (1982) Food intolerance: a major factor in the pathogenesis of irritable bowel syndrome. *Lancet* ii, 115–117.

Kagnoff, M.F. (1978a) Effects of antigen feeding on intestinal and systemic immune responses. I. Priming of precursor cytotoxic T cells by antigen feeding. *J Immunol* 120,395–399.

Kagnoff, M.F. (1978b) Effects of antigen feeding on intestinal and systemic immune responses. II. Suppression of delayed type hypersensitivity responses. *J Immunol* 120, 1509–1513.

Kagnoff, M.F. (1978c) Effects of antigen feeding on intestinal and systemic immune responses. III. Antigen-specific serum mediated suppression of humoral antibody responses after antigen feeding. *Cell Immunol* 40, 186–203.

Kagnoff, M.F. (1981) Immunological unresponsiveness after enteric antigen administration. In Strober, W. & Hanson, L.A. (eds), *Mucosal Immunity*, pp. 96–111. Raven Press, New York.

Kagnoff, M.F. (1982) Oral tolerance. *Ann N Y Acad Sci* 392, 248–264.

Kagnoff, M.F. & Campbell, S. (1976) Antibody dependent cell-mediated cytotoxicity; comparative ability of murine Peyer's patch and spleen cells to lyse lipopolysaccharide-coated and uncoated erythrocytes. *Gastroenterology* 70, 341–346.

Kawanishi, H., Saltzman, L.E. & Strober, W. (1983a) Mechanisms regulating IgA class specific immunoglobulin production in murine gut associated lymphoid tissues. I. T cells derived from Peyer's patches that switch sIgM B cells to sIgA B cells *in vitro. J Exp Med* 157, 433–450.

Kawanishi, H., Saltzman, L.E. & Strober, W. (1983b) Mechanisms regulating IgA class specific immunogobulin production in murine gut associated lymphoid tissues. II. Terminal differentiation of post-switch sIgA-bearing Peyer's patch B cells. *J Exp Med* 158, 649–669.

Keljo, D.J. & Hamilton, J.R. (1983) Quantitative determination of macromolecular transport rate across intestinal Peyer's patches. *Am J Physiol* 244, G637–G644.

Kenny, J.F., Boesman, M.I. & Michaels, R.H. (1967) Bacterial and viral copro-antibodies in breast-fed infants. *Pediatrics* 37, 202–213.

Kimpton, W.G., Washington, E.A. & Cahill, R.N.P. (1989) Recirculation of lymphocyte subsets (CD5+, CD4+, CD8+, SBU-T19+, and B cells) through gut and peripheral lymph nodes. *Immunology* 66, 69–75.

Krahenbuhl, J.P. & Campiche, M.A. (1969) Early stages of intestinal absorption of specific antibodies in the newborn. An ultrastructural, cytochemical, and immunological study in the pig, rat, and rabbit. *J Cell Biol* 42, 345–365.

Kurz, R., Mayr, J., Hofler, K.H., Falk, W. & Rosanelli, K. (1986) Immunologic findings in oral pertussis vaccination. *Padiatr Padol* 21, 53–59.

Lamont, A.G., Mowat, A.M. & Parrott, D.M.V. (1989) Priming of systemic and local delayed type hypersensitivity responses by feeding low doses of ovalbumin to mice. *Immunology* **66**, 595–99.

Lehmann, C.W. (1980) A double-blind study of sub-lingual provocation food testing: a study of its efficacy. The leukocytic food allergy test: a study of its reliability and reproducibility. Effect of diet and sublingual food drops on this test. *Ann Allergy* **45**, 144–149, 150–158.

Lessof, M.H., Wraight, D.G., Merrett, T.G. *et al.* (1980) Food allergy and intolerance in 100 patients. *Q J Med* **195**, 259–271.

MacDermott, R.P. & Bienenstock, J. (1979) Evidence for a common mucosal immunologic system. I-Migration of B immunoblasts into intestinal, respiratory, and genital tissues. *J Immunol* **122**, 1892–1897.

Mattingly, J.A. & Waksman, B.Y. (1978) Immunologic suppression after oral administration of antigen. I-Specific suppressor cells formed in rat Peyer's patches after oral administration of sheep erythrocytes and their systemic migration. *J Immunol* **121**, 1878–1883.

McGhee, J.R., Michalek, S.M., Kiyono, H., Babb, J.L., Clark, M.P. & Mosteller, L.M. (1982) Lipopolysaccharide of the IgA immune response. In Strober, W., Hanson, L.A., Sell, K.W. (eds), *Recent Advances in Mucosal Immunity*, pp. 57–72. Raven Press, New York.

McKee, A.M., Prior, A.M. & Whorwell, P.J. (1987) Exclusion diets in irritable bowel syndrome: are they worthwhile? *J Clin Gastroenterol* **9**, 526–528.

Middleton, E., Reed, C. & Ellis, E. (eds) (1983) *Allergy: Principles and Practice.* Mosby, St Louis.

Molkou, P. & Waguet, J.C. (1981) Food allergy and atopic dermatitis in children: treatment with oral sodium cromoglycate. *Ann Allergy* **47**, 173–175.

Nakagawa, T. & deWeck, A.L. (1983) Membrane receptors for the IgG_4 subclass human basophils and mast cells. *Clin Rev Allergy* **1**, 197–206.

Nanda, R., James, R., Smith, H., Dudley, C.R.K., Jewell, D.P. (1989) Food intolerance and the irritable bowel syndrome. **Gut** **30**, 1099–1104.

Ngan, J. & Kind, L.S. (1978) Suppressor T cells for IgE and IgG in Peyer's patches of mice made tolerant by the oral administration of ovalbumin *J Immunol* **120**, 861–865.

Ogra, P.L. & Karzon, D.T. (1969) Distribution of poliovirus antibody in serum, nasopharynx and alimentary tract following segmental immunization of lower alimentary tract with poliovaccine. *J Immunol* **102**, 1423–1430.

Ogra, S.S., Weintraub, D. & Ogra, P.L. (1977) Immunologic aspects of human colostrum and milk. III. Fat and absorption of cellular and soluble components in the gastrointestinal tract of the newborn. *J Immunol* **119**, 245–248.

O'Mahony, S., Arrantz, E., Barton, J.R. & Ferguson A. (1990a) Dissociation between systemic and mucosal humoral immune response in coeliac disease. *Gut* **32**, 29–35.

O'Mahony, S., Barton, J.R., Crichton, S. & Ferguson A. (1990) An appraisal of gut lavage in the study of intestinal humoral immunity. *Gut* **31**, 1341–1344.

Owen, R.L., Pierce, N.F., Apple, R.T. & Cray, W.C. Jr. (1986) M cell transport of *Vibrio cholerae* from the intestinal lumen into Peyer's patches: a mechanism for antigen sampling and for microbial transepithelial migration. *J Infect Dis* **153**, 1108–1118.

Pallone, F., Fais, S. & Capobianchi, M.R. (1988) HLA-D region antigens on isolated human colonic epithelial cells: enhanced expression in inflammatory bowel disease and *in vitro* induction by different stimuli. *Clin Exp Immunol* **74**, 75–79.

Pappo, J. & Owen, R.L. (1988) Absence of secretory component expression by epithelial cells overlying rabbit gut-associated lymphoid tissue. *Gastroenterology* **95**, 1173–1177.

Petit-Pierre, M., Gumowski, P. & Girard, J.P. (1985) Irritable bowel syndrome and hypersensitivity to food. *Ann Allergy* **54**, 538–540.

Pierce, N.F. (1978) The role of antigen form and function in the primary and secondary intestinal immune responses to cholera toxin and toxoid in rats. *J Exp Med* **148**, 195–206.

Reimann, H.J. & Lewin, J. (1988) Gastric mucosal reactions in patients with food allergy. *Am J Gastroenterol* **83**, 1212–1219.

Richman, L.K., Graeff, A.S. & Strober, W.S. (1981) Antigen presentation by macrophage-enriched cells from the mouse Peyers's patch. *Cell Immunol* **62**, 110–118.

Roberton, D.M., Paganelli, R., Dinwiddie, R. & Levinsky, R.J. (1982) Milk antigen absorption in the preterm and term neonate. *Arch Dis Child* **57**, 369–372.

Roberts, S.A., Reinhardt, M.C., Paganelli, R. & Levinsky, R.J. (1981) Specific antigen exclusion and non-specific facilitation of antigen entry across the gut in rats allergic to food proteins. *Clin Exp Immunol* **45**, 131–136.

Rothberg, R.M., Kraft, S.C. & Michalek, S.M. (1973) Systemic immunity after local antigenic stimulation of the lymphoid tissue of the gastrointestinal tract. *J Immunol* **111**, 1906–1913.

Royal College of Physicians (1984) Food intolerance and food aversion: a joint report of the Royal College of Physicians and the British Nutrition Foundation. *J Roy Coll Physicians Lond* **18**, 83–123.

Russell, D.A. & Castro, G.A. (1985) Anaphylactic-like reaction of small intestinal epithelium in parasitized guinea-pigs. *Immunology* **45**, 573–579.

Shiner, M., Ballard, J. & Smith, M.E. (1975) The small intestinal mucosa in cow's milk allergy. *Lancet* **i**, 136–138.

Smith, D.J. & Taubman, M.A. (1987) Oral immunization of humans with *Streptococcus sobrinus* glycosyltransferase. *Infect Immun* **55**, 2562–2569.

Smith, D.J., Gahnberg, L., Taubman, M.A. & Ebersole, J.L. (1986) Salivary antibody responses to oral and parenteral vaccines in children. *J Clin Immunol* **6**, 43–49.

Strobel, S., Busuttil, A. & Ferguson, A. (1983) Human intestinal mucosal mast cells: expanded population in untreated coeliac disease. *Gut* **24**, 222–227.

Swarbrick, E.T., Stokes, C.R. & Soothill, J. (1979) Absorption of antigens after oral immunization and simultaneous induction of specific systemic tolerance. *Gut* **20**, 121–125.

Taubman, M.A., Ebersole, J.L., Smith D.J. & Stack, W. (1983) Adjuvants for secretory immune responses. *Ann N Y Acad Sci* **409**, 637–49.

Taylor, B., Norman, A.P., Orgel, H.A., Stokes, H.R., Turner, J.W. & Soothill, J.F. (1973) Transient IgA deficiency and pathogenesis of infantile atopy. *Lancet* **ii**, 111–113.

Udall, J.N. & Allan Walker, A. (1987) Mucosal defence mechanisms. In Marsh, M.N. (ed), *Immunopathology of the Small Intestine*, pp. 11–17. Wiley, Chichester.

Wachsmann, D., Klein, J.P., Scholler, M. & Frank, R.M. (1985) Local and systemic immune response to orally administered liposome-associated soluble *S. mutans* cell wall antigens. *Immunology* **54**, 189–93.

Waldman, R.H., Stone, J., Bergmann, K.C. *et al.* (1986) Secretory antibody following oral influenza immunization. *Am J Med Sci* **292**, 367–71.

Wallach, D., Fellous, M. & Revel, M. (1982) Preferential effect of gamma-interferon on the synthesis of HLA antigens and their mRNAs in human cells. *Nature* **299**, 833–836.

Zwetchkenbaum, J.F. & Burakoff, R. (1988) Food allergy and the irritable bowel syndrome. *Am J Gastroenterol* **83**, 901–904.

13 Pathophysiological Mechanisms Associated with Type 1 Hypersensitivity Reactions in the Intestine

A.W. Cuthbert

INTRODUCTION

In a review of mechanisms by which antigens may precipitate type I hypersensitivity reactions in the sensitized gut it is wise to start with those things which are reasonably certain. Secretory diarrhoea, which can have a multitude of causes, is associated with a loss of salts, water and often glycoproteins from the intestinal wall into the lumen. It is important to realize that this is due mainly to an active secretory process often associated with a reduction of the absorptive processes for ions. Crucially it is an alteration in ion transporting activity which provides the local osmotic gradients for water loss into the intestine. While absorption of inorganic salts from the intestine is 'sodium led', the secretory process for ions is dependent on the active secretion of chloride ions. Obviously, the mass laws and those of electroneutrality mean that an equivalent number of cations and anions must be transported, either in absorption or secretion, but it is important to understand that the active transport of either an anion or a cation creates the appropriate electrical gradient for the movement of the counterion.

A further important feature of intestinal ion transport is that the processes of ion absorption and secretion generally take place in different cells, secretion being the activity expressed by the crypts while surface cells and villus epithelium are predominantly absorptive in character (Welsh *et al.*, 1982). There are a number of relatively detailed reviews of ion transport in the intestine to which the reader is referred, otherwise Fig. 13.1 illustrates some of the basic cellular mechanisms which are involved (Frizzell *et al.*, 1979; Donowitz & Welsh, 1986). In the villus cell sodium ions enter electrogenically, either alone through special channels which can be blocked with amiloride or along with organic solutes such as glucose or amino acids using carrier systems. Alternatively sodium ions enter the apical side along with chloride using a cotransporter. Whichever way sodium ions gain apical entry they are expelled by a pump (Na^+-K^+ ATPase) on the basolateral margin of the

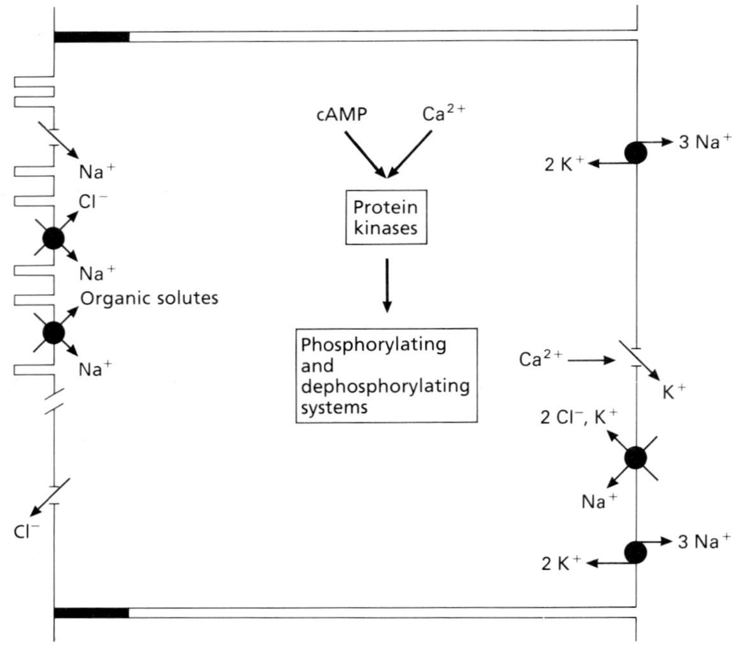

Fig. 13.1. Diagram of ion transport processes in a gut epithelial cell. The upper part of the figure represents a villus cell with apical microvilli. Na$^+$ ions enter the cell either via amiloride-sensitive Na$^+$ channels, a NaCl transporter or carrier systems along with sugars or amino acids. Na$^+$ is then eliminated from the cell by a sodium pump (Na$^+$-K$^+$-ATPase). In crypt cells chloride ions move uphill into the cell together with Na$^+$ and K$^+$ and leave through the apical membrane chloride channels. Again Na$^+$ is expelled by the basolateral sodium pump and K$^+$ equilibrates through basolateral K$^+$ channels. Interacting phosphorylation-dephosphorylation systems control the activity of membrane transport processes. The former are activated by protein kinases which themselves are dependent upon second messengers, particularly cAMP and Ca^{2+}. Additionally Ca^{2+} can activate basolateral K$^+$ channels.

cell, anions following passively via either an intracellular or a paracellular route. Thus the absorptive process is 'sodium led'.

In order to secrete chloride ions actively the crypt cells must accumulate chloride ions intracellularly to a level greater than that expected from the electrochemical gradients. To do this a triporter is used which carries two chloride ions accompanied by a sodium-ion and a potassium ion. Sodium ions can be expelled by the sodium pump, the source of energy for both secretory and absorptive processes, while the potassium ion can re-equilibrate across the potassium-permselective basolateral face of the cell. Then, if chloride channels are both present and open, chloride ions can exit from the apical surface, providing the appropriate electrical gradient for the movement of a counterion, usually sodium.

Turning now to aspects of epithelial ion transport which are less clearly worked out, we can consider how the various pumps, cotransporters, carriers and ion channels are regulated in a way which promotes or inhibits either absorption or secretion. Cells contain a regulatory network of interlinked protein phosphorylation and dephosphorylation events which control a huge variety of cellular processes. This network is regulated by a variety of protein kinases which are dependent upon cAMP, Ca-calmodulin or activation by diacylglycerol. These kinases therefore provide the link between the second messengers generated by recognition—transduction phenomena at the cell surface and the operation of mechanisms which alter cell function, in this instance alterations in the absorption or secretion of ions. In some circumstances details of these events have been worked out. For example, the open state probability of epithelial apical chloride channels is increased by cAMP or other agents which generate this second messenger (Welsh, 1986; Halm *et al.*, 1988). There are also many studies which show that the absorptive process for sodium chloride cotransport is inhibited in situations where cellular cAMP or indeed intracellular calcium ions are elevated (Racusen & Binder, 1977; Cuthbert, 1985). Thus, in consequence of either increased cellular cAMP and/or calcium, there is increased intestinal secretion and reduced absorption of ions, a preliminary to the secretory diarrhoeal state. One action of intracellular calcium which is well understood is that calcium sensitive potassium channels in the basolateral membrane are opened. As a result, potassium leak from the cells feeds the triporter system which promotes chloride uptake from the basolateral side. Furthermore the apical membrane of the epithelial cell hyperpolarizes (as indeed does the basolateral membrane), promoting chloride exit through apical channels.

The overwhelming reason for providing details of the transport processes in gut epithelium is that the mediators associated with immediate hypersensitivity reactions elevate either cellular cAMP or Ca_i (internal calcium ion concentration) and secretion is therefore set in motion. The rest of this chapter provides evidence for the hypothesis that local acute hypersensitivity reactions can take place in the gut, following sensitization and exposure to mundane antigenic stimuli such as everyday foodstuffs, intestinal parasites and the like.

THE EARLY MODEL

As chloride secretion is an electrogenic process, it can be monitored *in vitro* by voltage clamping a small sheet of epithelium at zero potential, i.e. short-circuiting.

The current recorded with time then represents charge transfer across the epithelium which can be converted to equivalents using the Faraday relationship. Of course it is necessary also to measure bi-directional ion fluxes using radioisotopes to discover which ions

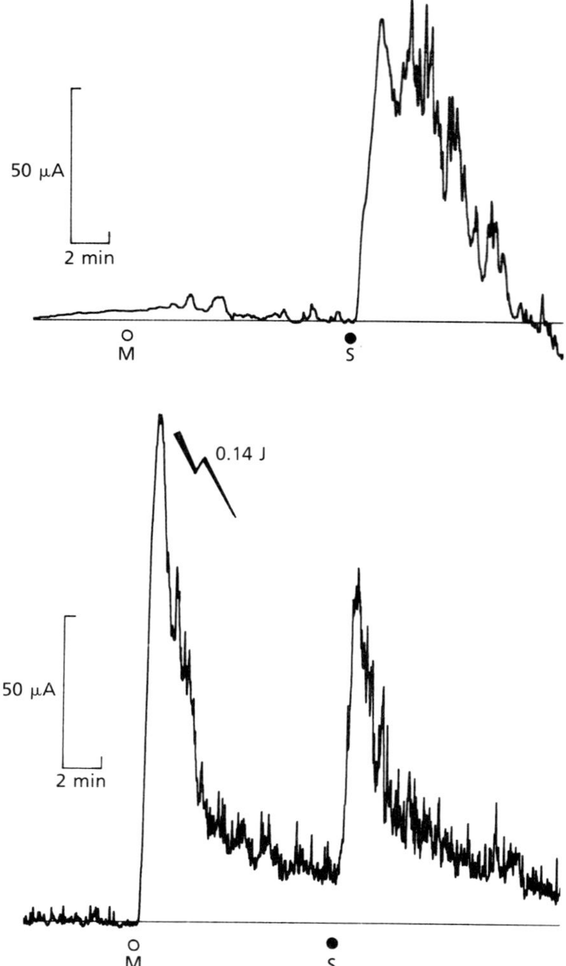

Fig. 13.2. SCC records for two colonic epithelial preparations (0.6 cm²) both from the same guinea-pig sensitized to BLG by drinking milk. Both preparations were challenged with BLG (10 μg ml⁻¹) first on the apical (○ M) and then the basolateral (● S) side. The preparation illustrated by the upper trace was otherwise untreated and did not respond to apical BLG. The lower trace illustrates a preparation which was first irradiated on the apical side with UV (0.14 J, 254 nm). This preparation now responded to both apical and basolateral BLG. Horizontal lines indicate zero SCC.

are transported and in which direction. Nevertheless the total net transfer of charge measured with the isotopes must be equivalent to the short-circuit current.

In the first study using this approach, the epithelia used were dissected from the colons of guinea-pigs which had been given cows' milk to drink rather than water, a protocol known to sensitize the animals to cow milk proteins. In a few initial experiments antigen challenge was with a few drops of milk, but in subsequent experiments bovine β-lactoglobulin (BLG) was used. Addition of either challenge caused an immediate and massive increase in short circuit current (SCC) when application was to the baso-lateral side of the tissue. The characteristics of the responses had all the qualities of an immediate hypersensitivity reaction as worked out in a series of subsequent studies. They were:

1 Challenge with BLG only gave responses in tissues from animals sensitized by milk drinking and not in water-drinking animals (Cuthbert *et al.*, 1983).

2 The response was around 10 times larger when the challenge was applied basolaterally than apically. Antigen (BLG) concentrations as small as 1 nmol could elicit responses (Cuthbert *et al.*, 1983).

3 Measurement of isotope fluxes and the use of drugs blocking chloride secretion indicated that the responses were due largely to a massive, inappropriate chloride secretion (Cuthbert *et al.*, 1983).

4 A similar sensitivity could be conveyed to non-sensitized colonic epithelia by exposing them to serum from sensitized animals (Cuthbert *et al.*, 1983).

It is quite clear therefore that it is possible to sensitize guinea-pigs to BLG by feeding milk orally and that when appropriately chal-lenged *in vitro* a cascade of events occurs which could underlie the secretory diarrhoeal state. However, as a model of food allergic disease there are some criticisms. First, the animals appeared per-fectly healthy when fed milk, and second, diarrhoea is more likely to result from excessive intestinal secretion such that if the absorp-tive ability of the colon is exceeded a diarrhoeal state ensues. Finally, *in vitro*, apical application of antigen is not very effective. These deficiencies in the model have been addressed in a series of other studies. First, by lesioning the apical surface of the colonic epithelium it was possible to elicit a maximal reaction with antigen applied to that face. A variety of lesioning methods were used such as UV irradiation (Kessel & Cuthbert, 1984), bile salts and detergents (Baird & Cuthbert, 1985) or simply time, i.e. to allow the preparations to remain *in vitro* for prolonged periods before challenge (Fig. 13.2).

These results suggest that not only is it necessary for cells of the immune systems to be sensitized, but that the provocation of a diarrhoeal attack on subsequent exposure is more likely when the defensive barrier of the gut is weakened. In this context it is of interest that cow's milk hypersensitivity in infants may often appear following bacterial gut infections (Gruskay & Cooke, 1955). Using an identical approach with intestinal epithelium in milk-fed guinea-pigs to that used for the colon, we found that similar immediate hypersensitivity reactions could be induced, although there were important differences to the colon (Baird *et al.*, 1984). These were:

1 BLG challenge from either the apical or basolateral face elicited a response. If a tissue was challenged first from the basolateral side

there was no subsequent response to apical challenge. The reverse of this was not so. Clearly the antigen needs to reach cells of the immune system located beneath the epithelium, a process more easily achieved with basolateral application.

2 There was an overall accumulation of fluid in the lumen in the absence of an osmotic gradient, indicating a secretion of ions towards the lumen. However it was not possible to identify the ion(s) involved by measuring fluxes of chloride and sodium ions. A combination of piretanide (a chloride transport blocker) and acetazolamide (a carbonic anyhydrase inhibitor), but neither alone, caused a significant inhibition of the response in the ileum. This contrasts with the colon where piretanide alone blocked the response, while acetazolamide was ineffective. This suggests, but has not been proved, that the guinea-pig ileum is a permissive epithelium in which either chloride or bicarbonate may be transported by the electrogenic secretory mechanism.

It needed to be established that the stimulation of electrogenic anion transport by adding antigen to sensitized guinea-pig epithelia was a general phenomenon applying also to other species and other antigens. Rat colonic epithelia from animals sensitized to ovalbumin showed similar SCC responses (Baird *et al.*, 1987). Oral challenge of rats sensitized to ovalbumin was shown by others to promote the accumulation of ^{125}I-labelled bovine serum albumin in intestinal tissue (Byars & Ferraresi, 1976) and to reduce the absorption of water and sodium and chloride ions from the lumen (Perdue *et al.*, 1984a). A fuller study with ovalbumin as antigen (Perdue & Grant Gall, 1986) has shown that the SCC responses are associated with electrogenic chloride secretion.

PARASITIC INFECTION AS A SENSITIZING MECHANISM

The rejection of nematode parasites by mammalian hosts is known to require the major components of the immune system (Ogilvie & Love, 1974). The rapid rejection of secondary infections suggests that a type I hypersensitivity reaction is involved (Miller *et al.*, 1981). This latter, together with the mast cell hyperplasia which results from infection (Miller, 1980), led us to investigate chloride secretion in isolated epithelium from infested animals. Rats were infected with the nematode *Nippostrongylus brasiliensis* and colonic epithelium dissected for SCC recording 30–40 days later. Challenge was with a mixture of nine body wall proteins prepared from the worms (Baird *et al.*, 1985). Indeed, colonic epithelia from parasitized animals did show an increase in SCC when challenged with worm antigen. The characteristics of the response are as follows:

1 Challenge with worm antigen was effective only when applied to

previously parasitized tissues and when applied to the basolateral, but not the apical, side.

2 Net chloride efflux was more than sufficient to account for the SCC responses.

3 Anti-rat IgE mimicked the effects of worm antigen and desensitized the tissue to its effect. Responses to anti-rat IgE were larger in sensitized animals than in controls, the difference representing, presumably, a greater degree of sensitization by IgE antibodies produced in response to worm antigens.

Concurrent investigations using guinea-pigs infected with *Trichinella spiralis* were reported by Russell (1986) and by Russell and Castro (1985). They showed that *Trichinella* proteins caused a chloride-dependent increase in SCC in jejunal epithelium from infected guinea-pigs and, importantly, that this sensitivity could be transferred passively to epithelium taken from non-infected animals.

Thus it is reasonably secure that infestation with nematode parasites sensitizes the gut epithelium of at least two species such that a type I hypersensitivity reaction ensues after exposure to body wall proteins from the parasites. Much has been written to suggest that the fluid secretion which flows from the crypts can flush away parasites attempting to re-establish an infection. However, this hypothesis is beyond the scope of this review.

MEDIATORS OF EPITHELIAL HYPERSENSITIVITY REACTIONS

There can be no doubt that the effect of antigen challenge in sensitized tissues is indirect, as in all the studies referred to so far the antigens had no effect on control tissues. However, it is much less clear which cells are sensitized following exposure to antigen and release the mediators which affect epithelial function. Clearly the mucosal mast cell is a serious candidate, since not only is there often a mucosal mast cell hyperplasia following sensitization, but isolated sensitized mucosal mast cells have been shown to release mediators following antigen challenge *in vitro*. Nevertheless there is an urgent need to demonstrate the localization of antigen under conditions which, *in vitro*, provoke an immediate hypersensitivity reaction. As well as cells within the lamina propria, the heterogenous group of cells known as intraepithelial leukocytes (Ernst *et al.*, 1985) are also potential candidates for involvement.

The actual nature of the mediators involved in type I hypersensitivity reactions in the gut have been derived from two types of study. In the first, various blocking agents have been used which either inhibit the actions of autacoids or prevent their release or generation. A more direct way is to measure the depletion of a putative autacoid following a type I reaction. This latter is fraught

Table 13.1. Mediators in intestinal anaphylaxis

Species and tissue	Sensitizing antigen	Mediators	Reference
β-lactoglobulin	Guinea-pig colon	Prostaglandins (indomethacin); histamine (mepyramine)	Cuthbert *et al.* 1983
β-lactoglobulin	Guinea-pig ileum	Atropine, mepyramine, disodium cromoglycate and indomethacin all ineffective	Baird *et al.* 1984
β-lactoglobulin	Guinea-pig ileum and colon	5HT (ICS 205 930)	Baird and Cuthbert, 1987
Ovalbumin	Rat ileum	Histamine (depletion)	Perdue *et al.* 1984a Perdue *et al.* 1984b
Ovalbumin	Rat jejunum	cAMP; response blocked by doxantrozole	Perdue and Grant-Gall 1986
Nippostrongylus brasiliensis	Rat colon	Mepyramine and indomethacin ineffective	Baird *et al.* 1985
Trichinella spiralis	Rat jejunum	Histamine (diphenhydyramine) prostaglandins (indomethacin)	Russell 1986
Trichinella spiralis	Rat jejunum	Release of 5HT, histamine and PGE$_2$	Castro *et al.* 1987

with difficulty as the responding cells may form only a small fraction of the tissue and the autacoid in question may not be exclusively contained in these cells. Table 13.1 summarizes present knowledge. It is clear that there is a variety of possible mediators which can be released, many of which may interact in concert either concurrently or consecutively to produce the overall effect. An interesting example of the interplay between mediators was given by Cuthbert and Baird (1986). Guinea-pig colon epithelium, sensitized to BLG, was mounted in chambers and challenged in the presence of 5 μmol/litre indomethacin. Some preparations were pre-incubated with either PGE$_2$ or PGD$_2$ (0.1 μmol/litre), concentrations which alone had no effect on SCC. Challenge with BLG gave responses (in μEq/10 minutes) of −0.04 in controls, 0.15 with PGE$_2$ and 0.24 with PGD$_2$. Thus in this system it appears that prostaglandins are vital for the response to be expressed. However, if prostaglandin (PG) synthesis is prevented then addition of eicosanoids, in concentrations which alone have no effect, restore the responsiveness to antigen. Thus the prostaglandins appear to act here in a permissive way.

ANTIGENS AND ANTIBODIES

The effect of different antigens in guinea-pigs sensitized by milk drinking was investigated using α- and β-lactoglobulin, casein, BSA and bovine γ-globulin. Only BLG showed substantial activity in relation to generating a type I response in epithelial tissues. However, both BLG and casein give PCA (passive cutaneous anaphylaxis) reactions in sensitized animals. It is of interest that BLG is the most foreign protein in cow's milk, being absent from the milk of humans and guinea-pigs (Baird *et al.*, 1984).

In rats sensitized with ovalbumin (Perdue *et al.*, 1984b) or infected with *Trichinella spiralis* (Harari *et al.*, 1987) the major antibody class associated with epithelial hypersensitivity was IgE. In guinea-pigs it was shown that purified IgG was able to transfer immediate hypersensitivity to colonic epithelium (Baird *et al.*, 1987).

INTRAMURAL NEURONES

The lamina propria of the intestine contains not only cells of the immune system along with connective tissue cells, blood vessels and the like but also neurones of the enteric nervous system. A number of chloride secretagogues cause their effects indirectly, apparently via actions on intramural neurones (Cooke & Carey, 1985). In two studies using epithelia from rat jejunum sensitized to *Trichinella spiralis* (Castro *et al.*, 1987) and guinea-pig ileum or colon sensitized to BLG (Baird & Cuthbert, 1987) the effect of challenge with antigen could be inhibited by tetrodotoxin, indicating that some part of the final effector mechanisms involved enteric neurones. These findings are of interest since an intimate anatomical association has been discovered between mucosal mast cells and peptidergic nerves (Stead *et al.*, 1987). Whether the communication is one- or two-way is not known. However, the combined effects of multiple mediators with neuronal modulation may mean that the genesis of the response to antigen may be very complex indeed. Castro *et al.* (1987) have shown the response occurs in two separate phases which they attribute to separate mediators.

STRUCTURAL CHANGES

Changes in ion transporting activity in sensitized tissues have been related temporally to diverse changes in the morphology of the tissue (Baron *et al.*, 1988). Guinea-pig epithelia sensitized to BLG were fixed 2 minutes after challenge; at the time the SCC response was maximal. Mucin expulsion from goblet cells of the crypts but not the villi occurred in the ileum, whereas goblet cells in the colon were insensitive to challenge. In the ileum the extracellular space in the lamina propria and intercellular space in the crypts diminished, while in the colon there was an eversion of the neck of the crypt onto the luminal surface. These morphological changes are probably not unique to hypersensitivity reactions as they are not dissimilar to changes reported with secretagogues such as lysylbradykinin (Baron *et al.*, 1986).

THE RECONSTRUCTED MODEL

From what has been discussed in the foregoing pages it is clear that epithelial hypersensitivity reactions in the gut are extremely complex. The epithelial preparation with the muscle layers removed is still a very complex tissue. An alternative way of investigating mechanisms is to reconstruct sensitized tissues from their component parts in order to discover which elements are responsible for generating which mediators. Baird *et al.* (1987) have reported a feasibility study along these lines. They constructed 'sandwiches' of human colonic epithelial cells with rat peritoneal mast cells. The mast cells were prepared either from control rats or from rats sensitized to ovalbumin. When challenged with antigen, 'sandwiches' containing sensitized mast cells responded with a chloride secretory response which was completely blocked by the H_1-receptor antagonist, mepyramine. For the future it will be possible to reconstruct tissues using only human cells. Separation of the various types of immune cells from human gut tissues will allow the role played by these cells alone and in combination to be assessed. Finally, it should not be impossible to culture epithelial cell monolayers upon a network of defined enteric neurones, so that the intriguing relationship between the nervous system and the immune system can be explored.

ACKNOWLEDGEMENTS

Work described here was supported by grants from Fisons plc, National Institutes of Health (HL 17705, F32-AM-07218-01) and the Nuffield Foundation.

REFERENCES

Baird, A.W. & Cuthbert, A.W. (1985) Changed sensitivity to antigen in a gut epithelium treated with bile salts. *Br J Pharmac* **84**, 653–656.

Baird, A.W. & Cuthbert, A.W. (1987) Neuronal involvement in type I hypersensitivity reactions in gut epithelia. *Br J Pharmac* **92**, 647–655.

Baird, A.W., Coombs, R.R.A., McLaughlan, P. & Cuthbert, A.W. (1984) Immediate hypersensitivity reactions to cow milk proteins in isolated epithelium from the ileum of milk-drinking guinea-pigs: comparisons with colonic epithelia. *Int Arch Allergy Appl Immun* **75**, 255–263.

Baird, A.W., Cuthbert, A.W. & Pearce, F.L. (1985) Immediate hypersensitivity reactions in epithelia from rats infected with *Nippostrongylus brasiliensis*. *Br J Pharmac* **85**, 787–795.

Baird, A.W., Cuthbert, A.W. & MacVinish, L.J. (1987) Type 1 hypersensitivity reactions in reconstructed tissues using syngeneic cell types. *Br J Pharmac* **91**, 857–869.

Baird, A.W., Barclay, W.S., Blazer-Yost, B.L. & Cuthbert, A.W. (1987) Affinity purified immunoglobulin G transfers immediate hypersensitivity to guinea-pig colonic epithelium *in vitro*. *Gastroenterology* **92**, 635–642.

Baron, D.A., Miller, D.H. & Margolius, H.S. (1986) Kinins induce rapid structural changes in colon concomitant with chloride secretion. *Cell Tissue Res* **246**, 589–594.

Baron, D.A., Baird, A.W., Cuthbert, A.W. & Margolius, H.S. (1988) Intestinal anaphylaxis: rapid changes in mucosal ion transport and morphology. *Am J Physiol* **254**, G307–G314.

Byars, N.E. & Ferraresi, R.W. (1976). Intestinal anaphylaxis in the rat as a model of food allergy. *Clin Exp Immunol* **24**, 352–356.

Castro, G.A., Harari, Y. & Russell, D. (1987) Mediators of anaphylaxis-induced ion transport changes in small intestine. *Am J Physiol* **253**. G540–G548.

Cooke, H.J. & Carey, H.V. (1985) Pharmacological analysis of 5-hydroxytryptamine actions on guinea-pig ileal mucosa. *Eur J Pharmacol* **111**, 329–337.

Cuthbert, A.W. (1985) Calcium-dependent chloride secretion in rat colon epithelium. *J Physiol* **361**, 1–17.

Cuthbert, A.W. & Baird, A.W. (1986) Multiple mediators of type 1 hypersensitivity reactions in epithelia. Letter to the Editor. *Am J Physiol* **251**, G443–444.

Cuthbert, A.W., McLaughlan, P. & Coombs, R.R.A. (1983) Immediate hypersensitivity reaction to β-lactoglobulin in the epithelium lining the colon of guinea-pigs fed cow's milk. *Int Archs Allergy Appl Immun* **72**, 34–40.

Donowitz, M. & Welsh, M.J. (1986) Ca^{2+} and cyclic AMP in regulation of intestinal Na, K and Cl transport. *Ann Rev Physiol* **48**, 135–150.

Ernst, P.B., Befus, A.D. & Bienenstock, J. (1985) Leukocytes in the intestinal epithelium: an unusual immunological compartment. *Immunology Today* **6**, 50–55.

Frizzell, R.A., Field, M. & Schultz, S.G., (1979) Sodium-coupled chloride transport by epithelial tissues. *Am J Physiol* **236**, F1–F8.

Gruskay, F.L. & Cooke, R.E. (1955) The gastrointestinal absorption of unaltered protein in normal infants and in infants recovering from diarrhoea. *Pediatrics* **16**, 763–769.

Halm, D.R., Rechkemmer, G.R., Schoumacher, R.A & Frizzell, R.A. (1988) Apical membrane chloride channels in a colonic cell line activated by secretory agonists. *Am J Physiol* **254**, C505–C511.

Harari, Y., Russell, D.A. & Castro, G.A. (1987) Anaphylaxis-mediated epithelial chloride secretion and parasite rejection in rat intestine. *J Immunol* **138**, 1250–1255.

Kessel, D. & Cuthbert, A.W. (1984) Sidedness of the reaction to β-lactoglobulin in sensitised colonic epithelia. *Int Archs Allergy Appl Immun* **74**, 113–119.

Miller, H.R.P. (1980) The structure, function and origin of mucosal mast cells. A brief review. *Biol Cell* **39**, 229–232.

Miller, H.R.P., Huntley, J.F. & Wallace, G.R. (1981) Immune exclusion and mucus trapping during the rapid expulsion of *Nippostrongylus brasiliensis* from primed rats. *Immunology* **44**, 419–429.

Ogilvie, B.M. & Love, R.J. (1974) Co-operation between antibodies and cells in immunity to a nematode parasite. *Transplant Rev* **19**, 147–169.

Perdue, M.H. & Grant-Gall, D. (1986) Intestinal anaphylaxis in the rat: jejunal response to *in vitro* antigen exposure. *Am J Physiol* **250**, G427–G431.

Perdue. M.H., Chung, M. & Grant-Gall, D. (1984a) The effect of intestinal anaphylaxis on gut function in the rat. *Gastroenterology* **86**, 391–397.

Perdue, M.H., Forstner, J.F., Roomi, N.W. & Grant-Gall, D. (1984b) Epithelial response to intestinal anaphylaxis in rats: goblet cell secretion and enterocyte damage. *Am J Physiol* **247**, G632–G637.

Racusen, L.C. & Binder, H.J. (1977) Alteration of large intestinal electrolyte transport by vasoactive intestinal polypeptide. *Gastroenterology* **73**, 790–796.

Russell, D.A. (1986) Mast cells in the regulation of intestinal electrolyte transport. *Am J Physiol* **251**, G253–262.

Russell, D.A. & Castro, G.A. (1985) Anaphylactic-like reaction of small intestinal epithelium in parasitized guinea-pigs. *Immunology* **54**, 573–579.

Stead, R.H., Tomioka, M., Quinonez, G., Simon, G.T., Felton, S.Y. & Bienenstock, J. (1987) Intestinal mucosal mast cells in normal and nematode-infected rat intestines are in intimate contact with peptidergic nerves. *Proc Natl Acad Sci USA* **84**, 2975–2979.

Welsh, M.J. (1986) The apical-membrane chloride channel in human tracheal epithelium. *Science* **232**, 1648–1650.

Welsh, M.J., Smith, P.L., Fromm, M. & Frizzell, R.A. (1982) Crypts are the site of intestinal fluid and electrolyte secretion. *Science* **218**, 1219–1221.

14 *Mast Cell Interactions with Smooth Muscle and Nerves in the Gut: Speculation on Mast Cell Modulation of Gastrointestinal Motility*

S.M. Collins

INTRODUCTION

Gastrointestinal motility is regulated by extrinsic and intrinsic neural influences, by hormones and by the inherent properties of smooth muscle of the gut. Alterations in motility may arise from perturbations in each of these control systems.

The observation that motility disturbances occur in the context of intestinal inflammation or allergy, taken in conjunction with the knowledge that mast cells release substances capable of influencing smooth muscle and enteric nerve function, raises the possibility that motility may be subject to regulation by the gut immune system.

The mast cell has traditionally been viewed in the context of its role in immediate hypersensitivity reactions. However, attention has recently focused on the relationship between mast cells and enteric nerves in the gut, raising the possibilities that mast cells respond to neural signals and that mast cells modulate neural activity in the gut. In addition, there is recent evidence that chemical injury or physical handling of the gut increases mast cell numbers in the neuromuscular layers. These findings introduce the mast cell as a potential modulator of gut motility in conditions other than those involving immediate hypersensitivity reactions.

In this chapter, I will address the role of the mast cell as a modulator of intestinal motility. I will explore mechanisms by which mast cells might influence the motility apparatus of the gut, and will discuss how this may impact on our understanding of the pathogenesis of gastrointestinal disorders including irritable bowel syndrome (IBS). I will not attempt to provide a review of the immunology or cell biology of the mast cell, and the reader is directed elsewhere for such information (Befus *et al.*, 1988).

EVIDENCE IMPLICATING MAST CELLS IN MOTILITY DISORDERS

To examine whether mast cells might influence motility, it is reasonable to first investigate whether motility disturbances occur in conditions associated with immediate hypersensitivity reactions in the gut. In man, food allergy is accompanied by symptoms such as vomiting, diarrhoea and cramping (May, 1976) that are highly suggestive of underlying motility disturbances.

Changes in peristaltic activity have been observed endoscopically following the direct application of food allergens to the gastric mucosa in atopic individuals (Romanski, 1986). Changes in motility have also been observed radiologically following oral challenge in milk-allergic patients (Liu *et al.*, 1975). The passage of barium through the proximal small intestine was more rapid for up to 8 hours following milk ingestion than after milk-free formula in seven allergic patients. Milk ingestion was also accompanied by gastrointestinal symptoms. The findings were not likely to be due to lactose intolerance, since similar radiological findings were observed following the ingestion of lactose-free casein hydrolysate in distilled water. There is a recent preliminary report of prolonged gastro-intestinal transit time in skin test-positive (Rast) patients with adverse reactions to food (Cavallini *et al.*, 1988). Intestinal transit, measured using the breath hydrogen test after lactulose, was prolonged in food-allergic patients maintained for 1 month on an unrestricted diet. If confirmed, these findings raise the possibility that antigen ingestion may induce long-term changes in gastro-intestinal motility.

Studies in animals support the clinical observations in allergic patients. In preruminant calves, feeding heated soya bean flour produced alterations in small intestinal myoelectrical activity (Sissons, 1982). In egg-albumin sensitized rats, intraluminal application of the antigen, but not placebo, caused changes in myoelectrical and motor activity recorded *in vivo* from the small intestine (Scott *et al.*, 1988). These changes consisted of abolition of the migrating motor complex and an increase in the frequency of clusters of aborally propagated contractions. Antigen challenge also resulted in diarrhoea. Responses occurred rapidly (mean 23 minutes) after antigen challenge and were associated with diarrhoea. The results were interpreted in terms of an IgE-mediated immediate hypersensitivity reaction, based on elevation of serum IgE in sensitized rats, and by extrapolation of previous demonstrations of passive cutaneous anaphylaxis (Perdue & Gall, 1986a, 1986b), changes in mucosal mast cell number and specific protease II levels in the mucosa (Patrick *et al.*, 1984) following antigen challenge in the same model.

In rats previously infected with the nematode parasite *Trichinella spiralis*, subsequent exposure to the parasite results in its rapid expulsion from the gut. This is accompanied by changes in motility, although the contribution of these changes to the expulsion process is not fully understood. Changes in myoelectrical activity occurred within 15 minutes of reinfection by *T. spiralis* larvae in sensitized rats, and consisted of a decrease in slow wave frequency, an increase in spiking activity, disruption of the interdigestive cycle of myoelectrical activity, and the appearance of migrating action potential complexes (Palmer & Castro, 1986). Because the responses were specific for *T. spiralis* in that they did not occur with another parasite *Eimeria niesculzi*, and because of their rapid onset, the motility changes were viewed as part of an immunologically based anamnestic response. Changes were also reported in the propulsive behaviour of intestinal segments from *T. spiralis*-sensitized rats following exposure to the parasite (Alizadeh *et al.*, 1986). It is likely that the motor response was mediated, at least in part, via smooth muscle and/or nerves in the gut wall since the segments were extrinsically denervated. Because the *Trichinella* model is characterized by increases in serum IgE and the development of intestinal mastocytosis, it seems reasonable to anticipate that the mast cell contributed to these changes by interacting with smooth muscle and/or enteric nerves.

IN VITRO STUDIES ON MAST CELL INTERACTIONS WITH INTESTINAL MUSCLE

The ability of intestinal muscle from sensitized animals to contract on exposure to antigen has long been recognized, and has formed the basis of the Schulz–Dale Reaction (Coulson, 1953). However, initial descriptions emphasized the use of this response as a bioassay for anaphylactic agents, and did not address the issue of mast cell involvement. Although this may have been implicit, it was not addressed directly until others showed that pretreatment of the tissue with Compound 48/80, a mast cell degranulating agent, prevented the antigen-induced muscle contraction (Joiner *et al.*, 1974).

Recent studies using *T. spiralis* infected rats have examined the interaction between mast cells and smooth muscle from the sensitized intestine. In this model, rats were infected with *T. spiralis* and allowed to recover for 35–85 days before being sacrificed. Isometric contraction of jejunal longitudinal muscle strips was recorded before and after adding crude *T. spiralis* antigen and other agents to the tissue bath (Fig. 14.1). This approach was combined with histological examination of the muscle for mast cells (Vermillion *et al.*, 1988).

Antigen caused a concentration-dependent contraction of muscle from sensitized but had no effect on the uninfected control rats. In *Trichinella*-sensitized rats, contraction did not occur following exposure to antigen from *Nippostrongylus brasiliensis*. These results implied an immunological mechanism. A role for homocytotropic antibody was implicated by the ability of rabbit anti-IgE serum to mimic antigen-induced contraction in muscle from sensitized rats, and by the ability of antigen to induce contraction in

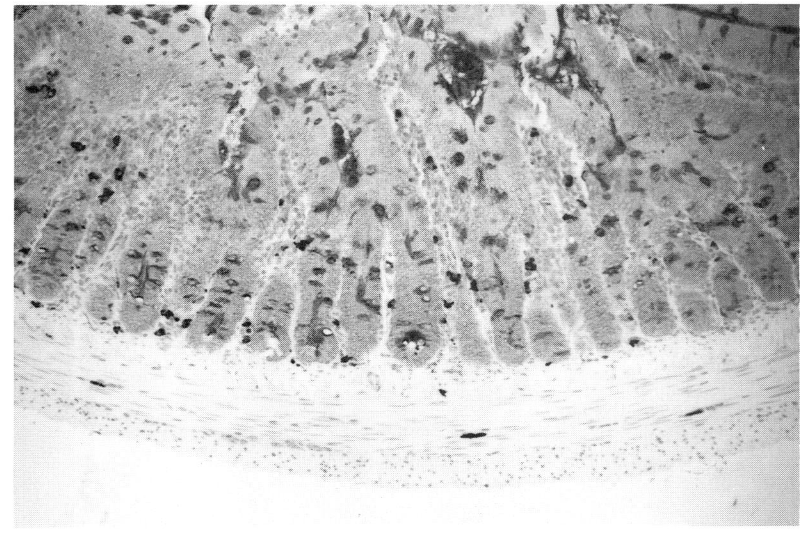

a

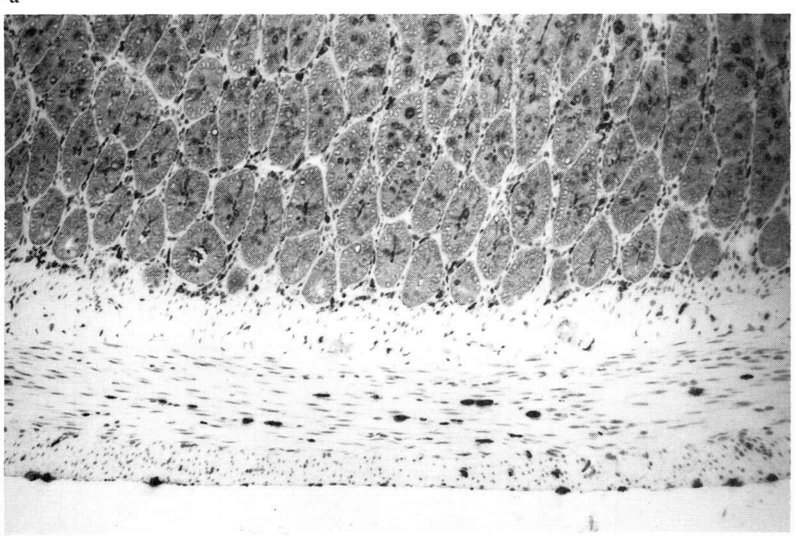

b

Fig. 14.1. Cross-sectional photomicrograph of jejunum from (a) control and (b) rat infected 55 days previously with *Trichinella spiralis*. Tissues fixed in Carnoy's and stained with toluidine blue. MC = mast cells. Note the increased numbers of mast cells in the muscle layers of the *Trichinella*-sensitized rat.

muscle from non-infected animals after preincubation of the muscle with serum from sensitized rats. The passive transfer phenomenon did not occur when the serum was heat-treated, again suggesting that IgE was involved.

Evidence that mast cells mediated the contraction was obtained from functional and histological studies. In muscle preincubated with a dose of antigen that would be expected to degranulate most of the mast cells present, subsequent addition of antigen resulted

Table 14.1. 5HT involvement in antigen-induced contraction in rat jejunum. Desensitization to 5HT was accomplished by exposing muscle strips to three cumulative additions of 1 µmol/l 5HT over a 60-minute period. Results shown are the mean ± SEM of at least four separate experiments, each involving three muscle strips

	Contraction (g/mm^2)
Antigen (1 µg/ml) alone	0.15 ± 0.07
Plus cyproheptidine (10 nmol/l)	0.05 ± 0.01
After 5HT desensitization	0.02 ± 0.01
Carbachol (1 µmol/l) alone	0.89 ± 0.20
Plus cyproheptidine	0.80 ± 0.20
After 5HT desensitization	0.84 ± 0.20

in little or no contractile response. In addition, the non-selective mast cell stabilizer doxantrazole, at a concentration that did not affect muscle contraction due to the muscarinic agonist carbachol, inhibited antigen-induced contraction. In muscle from sensitized rats, mast cell counts were increased 54-fold above controls. Following exposure to antigen, the number of identifiable mast cells in muscle from sensitized rats fell by 70%. These results are consistent with mast cell degranulation as a basis for antigen-induced muscle contraction.

Mast cells produce a variety of biologically active substances that are known to exert effects on intestinal nerve and muscle, and these include histamine, 5-hydroxytryptamine (5HT), prostaglandins, leukotrienes, and platelet activating factor (PAF; 1-0-alkyl-2-0-acetyl-sn-glycero-3-phosphorylcholine), in addition to several chemotactic factors (Marom & Castle, 1983). Mast cell-mediated contraction of muscle in the nematode-sensitized rat was mediated by 5HT. Contraction was inhibited by 5HT antagonists, cyproheptidine and following *in vitro* desensitization by 5HT, as shown in Table 14.1.

There was no effect of the histamine H$_1$ or histamine H$_2$ antagonists diphenhydramine and ranitidine, nor the prostaglandin synthetase inhibitor indomethacin (Vermillion *et al.*, 1988). The participation of other putative mediators such as leukotrienes or PAF in the antigen-induced response has not been evaluated. Since contraction occurred in the presence of tetrodotoxin, a direct interaction between 5HT and receptors on muscle cells was postulated.

Considerable evidence has emerged regarding the heterogeneity of mast cell populations (Enerbach, 1966; for review see Befus *et al.* 1986). Based on histochemical and pharmacological characteristics, mast cells have been classified into two main subpopulations, mucosal mast cells (MMCs) and connective tissue mast cells (CTMCs). The main points of distinction are summarized in Table 14.2.

Table 14.2. Characteristics of mast cell populations. A comparison of the histochemical and pharmacological properties of mucosal mast cells (MMCs), connective tissue mast cells (CTMCs) and mast cells (MC) studied *in situ* in intestinal muscle in the nematode-infected rat (from Vermillion *et al.*, 1988)

	MMC	CTMC	MC in gut muscle
Histochemistry			
Formalin sensitivity	+	0	
Positive alcian blue stain	+	0	
Positive safranine stain	0	+	
Specific protease	Type II	Type I	Type I
Proteoglycans	Chondroitin	Heparin	?
Pharmacology			
Antigen or anti-IgE	+	+	+
Concanavalin A	+	+	+
Compound 48/80	0	+	+
Substance P	+	+	?
Somatostatin	0	+	?
Neurotensin	0	+	?
VIP	0	+	?
Doxantrazole*	–	–	–
Cromoglycate[†]	0	–	–

* Able to stimulate histamine release from mast cells.
[†] Able to inhibit histamine release from mast cells.

Mucosal mast cells are found in submucosal regions in the lung and gut, and in the latter region these cells are now referred to as intestinal mucosal mast cells (IMMCs). CTMCs are found in a variety of tissues including the skin, tongue, lung parenchyma and lining the peritoneal cavity, from which they are easily isolated. Because of the ease with which CTMCs are isolated from the latter region, giving rise to a rapidly expanding literature, and in light of emerging differences between CTMCs in various tissues, the abbreviation PMC (peritoneal mast cell) has been used to identify those isolated from the peritoneum. It is important for the reader to appreciate that the field of mast cell heterogeneity is a rapidly advancing one in which further classification/subclassification is likely. It follows that one needs to be cautious in extrapolating characteristics obtained from mast cells in one tissue to those identified elsewhere, even though they belong to the same broad subpopulation based on the existing classification.

In the nematode model described above, studies to date have indicated that the mast cell in the longitudinal muscle of the intestine is of the connective tissue type. This is based on its staining properties with safranine and alcian blue (Wingren & Enerbach, 1983), and the presence of a distinct neutral type I protease (Lee *et al.*, 1985; Befus *et al.*, 1986). Functional evidence that these cells belong to the CTMC subpopulation is based on the demonstration that mast cell mediated muscle contraction may be induced by Compound 48/80 and inhibited by cromoglycate, substances believed to interact with CTMCs but not MMCs (Pearce *et al.*, 1982).

The determinants of mastocytosis in intestinal muscle in the nematode model have recently been addressed. Rats become sensitized to *T. spiralis* following the primary infection in which the jejunum is the primary habitat of adult worms. In the jejunum there is an inflammatory reaction involving the mucosa and submucosa but not the underlying tissues (Moqbel, 1986). However, smooth muscle and enteric nerve function is transiently altered in the jejunum (Collins *et al.*, 1988a; Vermillion & Collins, 1988a). Increases in mast cell number in the gut occur after expulsion of the nematode (Woodbury *et al.*, 1984). In muscle, mast cell numbers (expressed per unit cross sectional area of *muscle*), were greatest in the proximal small intestine and decreased in number along an aboral gradient down the gut (Collins *et al.*, 1988b). This suggests that local factors, most likely related to the primary infection, contribute to the development of mastocytosis in gut muscle. Whether this reflects a process initiated by the host or parasite remains to be determined.

The involvement of a systemic process in the development of mastocytosis in gut muscle is suggested by findings in muscle from jejunal segments *excluded* from the gut prior to oral infection with the parasite (Collins *et al.*, 1988b). Mast cell numbers were significantly greater in the excluded segments of infected rats compared to control. Similarly, *Trichinella* antigen contracted muscle only from excluded segments of sensitized rats. The mechanism underlying the increase in mast cell number in muscle from the worm-free excluded jejunal segment is not known and, again, could represent a sequence of events initiated by the parasite or the host. In muscle from the vas deferens of sensitized rats, which responded to exogenous 5HT, there was no contractile response to antigen and no increase in mast cell number, suggesting that the nematode-induced mastocytosis in smooth muscle is tissue specific. There was excellent correlation between mast cell number and the magnitude of contraction induced by antigen in excluded or retained gut muscle from sensitized rats when data were corrected for regional differences in muscle responsiveness to 5HT, the identified mediator of mast cell-induced contraction. However, a point of interest arises from the observation that mast cell numbers in colonic muscle from sensitized rats were not greater than those observed in control rats in other regions, yet contraction occurred with antigen or Compound 48/80 only in sensitized rats and was doxantrazole-sensitive. This finding raises the possibility that existing mast cells amplify smooth muscle responses by: (a) increasing the coupling of muscle in the vicinity of the mast cell; (b) causing neurotransmitter release; or (c) releasing substances that have a potentiating effect on stimuli arising from other cells, such as nerves or eosinophils.

INTERACTIONS BETWEEN MAST CELL AND ENTERIC NERVES

Structural and functional studies illustrate the feasibility of mast cell interactions with enteric nerves in the gastrointestinal tract. Several studies have demonstrated a close association between mast cells and nerves in the gut (Heine & Forster, 1975; Newson *et al.*, 1983; Yonei *et al.*, 1985; Stead *et al.* 1987) of several animal species, and also in patients with Crohn's Disease (Dvorak *et al.*, 1980).

In a recent study in the rat infected with the nematode parasite *Nippostrongylus brasiliensis*, Stead *et al.* (1987) found that the majority of the mast cells in the intestinal mucosa were in close proximity with nerves, many of which were substance P-containing nerves. In some instances, electron microscopy suggested direct membrane contact between the two cell types. This observation is supported by recent electrophysiological evidence of low-resistance communications between mast cells and nerves in a co-culture system (Blennerhassett *et al.*, 1987).

Functional evidence of mast cell influences on enteric nerves in the gut is based largely, but not exclusively, on indirect studies in the epithelium of sensitized animals. Models include rats or guinea-pigs infected with the nematodes *N. brasiliensis* or *T. spiralis*, or sensitized to ovalbumin or lactoglobulin. In these studies, exposure of epithelium to antigen resulted in changes in short-circuit current that were inhibited by the mast cell stabilizer doxantrazole or by the neuronal blocking agent tetrodotoxin (Perdue & Gall, 1986a,b; Baird & Cuthbert, 1987; Castro *et al.*, 1987), consistent with a mast cell-mediated effect on mucosal nerves. These studies have provided a basis for examining mast cell interactions with nerves in the myenteric plexus.

In the *Trichinella* sensitized rat model there is morphological evidence of mastocytosis in the myenteric plexus, with 5HT-containing mast cells in juxtaposition with nerve fibres (M. Blennerhassett, personal communication). There is preliminary data illustrating functional interactions between mast cells and type 2/AH neurones of the myenteric plexus in the *Trichinella spiralis*-sensitized guinea-pig (Palmer *et al.*, 1988). Exposure of the tissue to *Trichinella* antigen induced slow excitation characterized by membrane depolarization, increased input resistance, increased action potential discharge and a decreased amplitude of post-spike hyperpolarization. Taken together, these results provide structural and functional evidence in support of the concept that mast cells modulate function in the myenteric plexus.

The concept that enteric nerves influence mast cell function is attractive, but direct evidence in support of this is awaited (see Bienenstock, 1989; Stead *et al.*, 1989). Several neuropeptides have been shown to stimulate non-cytotoxic release of histamine from rat peritoneal mast cells (Piotrowski & Foreman, 1985; Shanahan *et al.*, 1985). Substance P, somatostatin, vasoactive intestinal polypeptide (VIP) and neurotensin produced a concentration-dependent increase in histamine release from PMCs. The concentrations required to induce these effects were high (0.1µmol/litre to 0.1 mmol/litre), but might be achieved *in situ* over the small distance that exists between mast cells and nerves in the gut. There is evidence obtained *in situ* to support neuromodulation of mast cell function. Bani-Sacchi *et al.* (1986) showed that parasympathetic nerve stimulation (10–20 Hz) increased the release of histamine from rat ileum, and this was considered to originate from mast cells because it was accompanied by a diminution of mast cell granule metachromasia. Since the effect was inhibited by tetrodotoxin or atropine, the authors concluded that there is modulation of mast cell function by parasympathetic nerves in the gut. This is supported by other studies demonstrating changes in granulated mast cell number in rat stomach after truncal vagotomy (Ganguly *et al.*, 1979). A previous study by Gerner *et al.* (1979) showed that the effect of cholecystokinin (CCK) on motor activity in the guinea-pig stomach was inhibited by mepyramine, suggesting mast cell involvement. However, this was not verified histologically or functionally using selective mast cell stabilizers. Thus, there is clearly sufficient data upon which to construct a viable hypothesis regarding the ability of the nervous system to alter motility through effects on the mast cell; however, formal experimental validation is required.

Table 14.3. Conditions associated with mastocytosis. Examples of clinical conditions and presumed underlying pathophysiological processes in which there are increased numbers of mast cells (adapted from Befus *et al.* 1986, with permission)

Condition	Process
Crohn's disease	
Ulcerative colitis	
Diverticular disease	Inflammation
Coeliac disease	
Graft vs. host disease	
Nematode infection	
Allergy (rhinitis, etc.)	Hypersensitivity
Scleroderma	
Scar tissue (keloid)	Injury and repair
Nerve damage	
Solid tumours	Neoplasia
Mastocytosis	

OTHER POTENTIAL LOCI FOR MAST CELL MODULATION OF MOTILITY

Gastrointestinal motility is subject to regulation via the release of gastrointestinal peptides from endocrine cells in the gut. It is possible that mast cells modulate motility by influencing the release of such peptide hormones as gastrin, CCK, etc. As suggested above, mast cells may also influence the coupling of smooth muscle by influencing the formation of gap junctions between cells, or by altering the pacemaker function of interstitial cells of Cajal. These possibilities require formal experimental evaluation.

DETERMINANTS OF MASTOCYTOSIS

Increased numbers of mast cells are found in the gut in a wide variety of clinical conditions, summarized in Table 14.3. These conditions reflect diverse pathological processes that include tissue repair and neoplasia in addition to inflammation and immediate (type I) hypersensitivity.

Studies in the rat have investigated stimuli for mast cell increases in the muscle layers of the gut, and results show that mastocytosis occurs in conditions other than nematode infection. Serosal application of the cationic surfactant benzalkonium chloride (BAC), a process reported to ablate the myenteric plexus (Fox *et al.*, 1983), caused a substantial increase in mast cell number in the outer layer of the longitudinal muscle and in the region of the myenteric plexus (Vermillion *et al.*, 1988b). Although BAC has been reported to inhibit histamine release from rat peritoneal mast cells, it is likely that the mastocytosis induced by BAC is a result of nerve damage. This interpretation is based on previous demonstrations that nerve injury by transection or a neuropathic process results in an increase in mast cell number (Olsson, 1968), an effect that may be related to the ability of nerve growth factor, released on nerve injury, to stimulate mast cell degranulation and growth *in vitro* (Aloe & Levi-Montcini, 1977; Bruni *et al.*, 1982).

An unanticipated but potentially important finding in the study by Vermillion and Collins (1988b) was that mast cell numbers increased in segments that had received saline administered by droplet or by rubbing a swab on the serosal surface 1 month previously. Since the increases were greater following swab application, we consider mechanical irritation to be a causative factor in the development of mastocytosis in gut muscle under these experimental conditions. Moreover, pretreatment of the animal with the CTMC stabilizer cromoglycate reduced the increase in mast cell numbers induced by saline application. This observation is supportive of the concept that mast cell degranulation product(s) stimulate mast cell proliferation (Enerbach & Lowhagen, 1979;

Marshall *et al.*, 1987). The extent to which this occurs in the human intestine, and its implications for the effects of surgical handling of the bowel on motility, remain a matter of speculation.

SPECULATION ON MAST CELL INVOLVEMENT IN GASTROINTESTINAL DISORDERS ASSOCIATED WITH ALTERED MOTILITY

Inflammatory bowel disease

The putative role of mast cells in the pathophysiology of idiopathic inflammatory bowel disease (IBD) has received considerable attention. There are increased numbers of mast cells in the gut of patients with ulcerative colitis or Crohn's disease, and there is evidence of degranulation when the disease is active (Heatley *et al.*, 1975a, 1975b). These findings, taken in conjunction with reports of symptomatic improvement in selected IBD patients following therapy with cromoglycate, a mast cell stabilizer (Heatley *et al.*, 1975a; Dronfield & Langman, 1978), suggest the involvement of mast cells in the pathophysiology of these disorders. Since ultrastructural studies have demonstrated degranulating mast cells in the vicinity of nerves and smooth muscle cells (Dvorak *et al.*, 1980), it is possible that mast cells contribute to altered motility seen in patients with active IBD (Kern *et al.*, 1951; Chaudhary & Truelove, 1961; Connell, 1962; Snape *et al.*, 1980).

Irritable bowel syndrome

There are several observations which, when taken together with the above-described information regarding mast cell interactions with nerves and muscle in the gut, prompt speculation on a potential role for the mast cell in the pathophysiology of IBS.

Tricyclic antidepressants, which have been shown to be of benefit to some IBS patients (Greenbaum *et al.*, 1987), are also known to influence mast cell function (Theoharides *et al.*, 1982). Increased intestinal prostaglandin production following double-blind exposure to certain foods in diarrhoea-predominant IBS patients with specific food intolerance raises questions regarding a possible immunological or inflammatory component to the pathophysiology of a subset of this syndrome (Jones *et al.*, 1982). The development of IBS in patients recovering from enteric infections (Chaudhary & Truelove, 1962) is also in keeping with an immunological or inflammatory mechanism in at least a subset of the IBS population. Studies in animals indicate that a mucosal inflammatory infiltrate in the gut increases the responsiveness of the underlying smooth muscle (Vermillion & Collins, 1988a), providing a possible link between intestinal inflammatory processes and increased motor responses. This may have a bearing on the exaggerated motor responses observed in IBS patients following pharmacological stimulation (Chaudhary & Truelove, 1961; Harvey & Read, 1973). Finally, the recent observation that IBS patients have hyper-responsive airways when challenged with methacholine invites comparisons between IBS and asthma—a condition in which interest has focused on mast cells, inflammation and altered smooth muscle function (Hargreaves *et al.*, 1986). What is now required is a formal assessment of mast cell presence and function in the gut wall of patients with IBS. To my knowledge, there is only one study that has examined mast cell numbers in functional bowel disease. In that study, marked increases in mast cell numbers were observed in colonic muscle from four patients with spastic colitis—a term often used to imply IBS (Hiatt & Katz, 1977).

Other gastrointestinal disorders

Increased numbers of mast cells have been demonstrated in sclero-derma, coeliac disease, diverticular disease (Hiatt & Katz, 1977) and graft vs. host disease. Clinical or radiological studies suggest altered motility patterns in these disorders, but the extent to which mast cells contribute to these changes remains to be determined.

CONCLUSIONS

Our perception of the mast cell is changing from one in which it was viewed almost entirely in the context of its involvement in immediate hypersensitivity reactions, to a new position in which the mast cell may be seen to play a modulatory role in physiological as well as immunological function. In that capacity, the mast cell may also be viewed as interfacing between the environment (via the immune system), the brain (via its interactions with nerves), and the major effector systems of the gut, including the motor apparatus.

In this chapter, I have tried to bring together information from a variety of sources to demonstrate the ability of the mast cell to interact with the motor system of the gut. It is hoped that this will provide an infrastructure upon which to base new approaches to the investigation of gastrointestinal disease characterized by motility disturbances for which there is no structural cause.

ACKNOWLEDGEMENTS

The author acknowledges Dr Dianne Vermillion, whose work has provided many of the experimental observations regarding mast cell interactions with smooth muscle in the gut. The author also thanks Ms Patricia Blennerhassett for her hard work, and Dr M. Blennerhassett for providing the photomicrograph. Dr Collins is supported by a grant from The Medical Research Council (MRC) of Canada.

Alizadeh, H., Weems, W.A. & Castro, G.A. (1986) Immunologically induced alterations in the intrinsic propulsive state of guinea pig jejunum *Gastroenterology* **91**, A1042 (abstract).

Aloe, L. & Levi-Montcini, R. (1977) Mast cells increase in tissues of neonatal rats injected with the nerve growth factor. *Brain Res* **133**, 358–366.

Baird, A.W. & Cuthbert, A.W. (1987) Neuronal involvement in type I hypersensitivity reactions in gut epithelia. *Brit J Pharmacol* **92**, 647.

Bani-Sacchi, T., Barattini, M., Bianchi, S. *et al.* (1986) The release of histamine by parasympathetic stimulation in guinea-pig auricle and rat ileum. *J Physiol* **371**, 29–43.

Befus, A.D., Bienenstock, J. & Denburg, J. (1986) *Mast Cell Differentiation and Heterogeneity*. Raven Press, New York.

Befus, A.D., Lee, T.D.G. & Bienenstock, J. (1988) Immunological and physiological features of mast cell functions of mucosal surfaces. Infections at mucosal surface. In Strober, W., Lemm, M.E. & McGhee, J. (eds), *Mucosal Immunity*, pp. 209–224. Oxford University Press, New York.

Bienenstock, J. (1989) An update on mast cell heterogeneity including comments on mast cell/nerve relationships. *J Allergy Clin Immunol* **81**, 763–769.

Blennerhassett, M.G., Stead, R.H. & Bienenstock, J. (1987) Association and interaction between sympathetic neurons and mast cells *in vitro*. *Biophysical J* **51**, 65A.

Bruni, A., Bigion, E., Boarato, E., Mieetto, L., Leon, A. & Toffano, G. (1982) Interaction between nerve growth factor and lysophosphotidylserine on rat peritoneal mast cells. *FEBS Lett* **138**, 190–192.

Castro, G.A., Havari, Y. & Russell, D. (1987) Mediators of anaphylaxis-induced ion transport changes in small intestine. *Am J Physiol* **253**, G540–548.

Cavallini, G., Barba, A., Riela, A. *et al.* (1988) Adverse food reaction and gastrointestinal transit time: a possible link. *Gastroenterology* **94**(2), A63.

Chaudhary, N.A. & Truelove, S.C. (1961) Human colonic motility: a comparative study of normal subjects, patients with ulcerative colitis and patients with irritable colon syndrome. II. Effect of prostigmine. *Gastroenterology* **40**, 18–26.

Chaudhary, N.A. & Truelove, S.C. (1962) The irritable colon syndrome. *Q J Med* **123**, 307–322.

Collins, S.M., Blennerhassett, P., Vermillion, D.L. & Blennerhassett, M. (1988a) *Trichinella spiralis* infection in the rat alters acetylcholine release from the myenteric plexus. *Gastroenterology* **94** (5), A74.

Collins, S.M., Marzio, L., Vermillion, D.L., Blennerhassett, P. & Chiverton, S. (1988b) The immunodulation of gut motility: factors that determine the proliferation of mast cells in the sensitized gut. *Gastroenterology* **94** (5) A75.

Connell, A.M. (1962) The motility of the pelvic colon. Part II. Paradoxical motility in diarrhea and constipation. *Gut* **3**, 342–348.

Coulson, E.J. (1953) The Schultz–Dale technique. *J Allergy* **24**, 458–473.

Dronfield, M.W. & Langman, M.J.S. (1978) Comparative trial of sulphasalazine and oral sodium cromoglycate in the maintenance of remission in ulcerative colitis. *Gut* **19**, 1136–1139.

Dvorak, A.M., Monahan, R.A., Osage, J.E. & Dickersin, G.R. (1980) Crohn's disease: transmission electron microscopic studies. II. Immunologic inflammatory response. Alterations in mast cells, basophils, eosinophils and the microvasculature. *Human Path* **11** (6), 606–619.

Enerbach, L. (1966) Mast cells in the gastrointestinal mucosa. I. Effects of fixation. *Acta Path Microbiol Scand* **66**, 289–302.

Enerbach, L. & Lowhagen, G.B. (1979) Long term increase in mucosal mast cells in rat induced by Compound 48/80. *Cell Tiss Res* **198**, 209–215.

Fox, D.A., Epstein, M.L. & Bass, P. (1983) Surfactants selectively ablate enteric neurons of the rat jejunum. *J Pharm Exp Therap* **227**, 538–544.

Ganguly, A.K., Sathiamoorthy, S.S. & Bhatnagar, O.P. (1979) Effect of subdiaphragmatic vagotomy on gastric mucosal mast cell population in pylorus-ligated rats. *Q J Exp Physiol* 63, 89.

Gerner, T., Haffner, J.F.W. & Norstein, J. (1979) The effects of mepyramine and cimetidine on the motor responses to histamine, cholecystokinin and gastrin in the fundus and antrum of isolated guinea-pig stomachs. *Scand J Gastroent* 14, 65–72.

Greenbaum, D.S., Mayle, J.E., Vanegeren, L.E. (1987) Effects of desipramine on irritable bowel syndrome compared with atropine and placebo. *Dig Dis Sci* 32, 257–266.

Hargreaves, F.E., Dolovitch, J., O'Byrne, P.M., Ramsdale, E.H. & Dankz, E.E. (1986) The origin of airway hyperresponsiveness. *J Allergy Clin Immunol* 78 (5), 825–832.

Harvey, R.F. & Read, A.E. (1973) The effect of cholecystokinin on colonic motility and symptoms in patients with the irritable colon syndrome. *Lancet* i, 1–3.

Heatley, R.V., Calcraft, B.J., Rhodes, E.O., Owen, E. & Evans, B.K. (1975a) Disodium cromoglycate in the treatment of chronic proctitis. *Gut* 16, 559–563.

Heatley, R.V., Rhodes, J., Calcraft, B.J., Whitehead, R.H., Fifield, R. & Newcombe, R.G. (1975b) Immunoglobulin E in rectal mucosa of patients with proctitis. *Lancet* 2, 1010–1012.

Heine, H. & Forster, F.I. (1975) Relationships between mast cells and preterminal nerve fibres. *Z. Mikrosk Anat Forsch Leipzig* 89, S934–937.

Hiatt, R.B. & Katz, J. (1977) Mast cells in inflammatory conditions of the gastro-intestinal tract. *Am J Gastroenterol* 37, 541–545.

Joiner, P.D., Wall, M., Davis, L.B. & Hahn, R. (1974) Role of amines in anaphyl-actic contraction of guinea-pig isolated smooth muscle. *J Allergy Clin Immunol* 53 (5), 261–270.

Jones, A.V., McLaughlan, P., Shorthouse, M., Workman, E. & Hunter, J.O. (1982) Food intolerance: a major factor in the pathogenesis of irritable bowel syndrome. *Lancet* ii, 1115–1117.

Kern, F., Almy, T.P., Abbot, F.K. & Bogdonoff, M.D. (1951) The motility of the distal colon in non-specific ulcerative colitis. *Gastroenterology* 19, 492–503.

Lee, T.D.G., Swieter, M., Bienenstock, J. & Befus, A.D. (1985) Heterogeneity in mast cell populations. *Clin Immunol Rev* 4, 143–199.

Liu, H-Y., Whitehouse, W.M. & Giday, Z. (1975) Proximal small bowel transit pattern in patients with malabsorption induced by bovine milk protein ingestion. *Radiology* 115, 415–420.

Marom, Z. & Castle, T.B. (1983) Mast cells and their mediators. *Ann Allergy* 50, 367–370.

Marshall, J., Prout, S.J., Jaffery, G. & Bell, E.B. (1987) Induction of an auto-anti-IgE response in rats. II. Effects on mast cell populations. *Eur J Immunol* 17, 445–451.

May, C.D. (1976) Objective clinical and laboratory studies of immediate hyper-sensitivity reactions to foods in asthmatic children. *J Allergy Clin Immunol* 50, 500.

Moqbel, R. (1986) Helminth-induced intestinal inflammation. *Trans Roy Soc Trop Med* 80, 719.

Newson, B., Dahlstrom, A., Enerbach, L. & Ahlman, H. (1983) Suggestive evidence for a direct innervation of mucosal mast cells. An electron microscopic study. *Neuroscience* 10, 565–570.

Olsson, Y. (1968) Mast cells in the nervous system. *Int Rev Cytol* 29, 27–70.

Palmer, J.M. & Castro, G.A. (1986) Anamnestic stimulus-specific myoelectrical responses associated with intestinal immunity in the rat. *Am J Physiol* 250, G266–273.

Palmer, J., Tamura, K. & Wood, J.D. (1988) Electrical and synaptic properties of myenteric plexus neurons from guinea pig small intestine during infection with *Trichinella spiralis. FASEB J* 2 (4), A325.

Patrick, M.K., Dunn, I.J., Buret, A. *et al.* (1984) Mast cell protease release and mucosal ultrastructure during intestinal anaphylaxis in the rat. *Gastroenterology* 86, 391–397.

Pearce, F.L., Befus, A.D., Gauldie, J. & Bienenstock, J. (1982) Mucosal mast cells. II. Effects of anti-allergic compounds on histamine secretion by isolated intestinal mast cells. *J Immunol* **128**, 2481–2486.

Perdue, M.H. & Gall, D.G. (1986a) Intestinal anaphylaxis in the rat: jejunal response to *in vitro* antigen exposure. *Am J Physiol* **250**, G427–431.

Perdue, M.H. & Gall, D.G. (1986b) Rat jejunal mucosal response to histamine and antihistamines *in vitro*. Comparison with antigen-induced changes during intestinal anaphylaxis. *Agents Actions* **19**, 5–9.

Piotrowski, W. & Foreman, J.C. (1985) On the actions of substance P, somatostatin and vasoactive intestinal polypeptide on rat peritoneal mast cells and in human skin. *Naunyn-Schmeidebergs Arch Pharmacol* **331**, 364–368.

Romanski, B. (1986) The pathology of food allergy studied by gastric allergen challenge. In Brostoff, J. & Challacombe, S.J. (eds), *Food Allergy*, pp. 917–930. Baillière Tindall, London.

Scott, R.B., Diamant, S.C. & Gau, D.G. (1983) Motility effects of intestinal anaphylaxis in the rat. *Am J Physiol* **255**, G505–G511.

Shanahan, F., Denburg, J.A., Fox, J., Bienenstock, J. & Befus, D. (1985) Mast cell heterogeneity: effects of neuroenteric peptides on histamine release. *J Immunol* **135**, 1331–1337.

Sissons, J.W. (1982) Effects of soya bean products on digestive processes in the gastrointestinal tract of preruminant calves. *Proc Nutr Soc* **41**, 53–60.

Snape, W.J. Jr., Matarazzo, S.A. & Cohen, S. (1980) Abnormal gastrocolic response in patients with ulcerative colitis. *Gut* **21**, 392–396.

Stead, R.H., Tomioka, M., Quinonez, G., Simon, G.T., Felten, S.Y. & Bienenstock, J. (1987) Intestinal mucosal mast cells in normal and nematode infected rat intestines are in intimate contact with peptidergic nerves. *Proc Natl Acad Sci USA*, **84**, 2975–2979.

Stead, R.H., Perdue, M.H., Blennerhassett, M.G., Kakuta, Y., Sestini, P. & Bienenstock, J. (1989) The innervation of mast cells. In Freoer, S. (ed), *Neuroendocrine–immune Network*, pp. 19–37. CRC Press, Boca Raton.

Theoharides, T.C., Bondy, P.K., Tsakalos, N.D. & Askenase, P.W. (1982) Differential release of serotonin and histamine from mast cells. *Nature* **297**, 229–231.

Vermillion, D.L. & Collins, S.M. (1988a) Increased responsiveness of jejunal longitudinal muscle in *Trichinella spiralis* rats. *Am J Physiol* **254**, G124–129.

Vermillion, D.L. & Collins, S.M. (1988b) Non-specific induction of mastocytosis in rat intestinal muscle. *Gastroenterology* **94**, A479.

Vermillion, D.L., Ernst, P.B., Scicchitano, R. & Collins, S.M. (1988) Antigen-induced contraction of jejunal smooth muscle in the sensitized rat. *Am J Physiol* **255**, G701–708.

Wingren, U. & Enerbach, L. (1983) Mucosal mast cells of the rat intestine: a re-evaluation of fixation and staining properties. *Histochem J* **15**, 571.

Woodbury, R.G., Miller, H.R.P., Huntley, G.F.J., Palliser, A.C. & Wakelin, D. (1984) Mucosal mast cells are functionally active during spontaneous expulsion of intestinal nematodes in the rat. *Nature* **312**, 450.

Yonei, Y., Oda, M., Nakamura, M. *et al.* (1985) Evidence for direct interaction between the cholinergic nerve and mast cells in rat colonic mucosa. An electron microscopic, cytochemical and autoradiographic study. *J Clin Electron Microsc* **18**, 560–561.

15 Systemic Mastocytosis and Regional Gastrointestinal Mast Cell Disease

P.B. Miner Jr

INTRODUCTION

The mast cell was discovered over 100 years ago on the basis of the metachromatic staining properties of the prominent cytoplastic granules. When first discovered, the mast cell was felt to produce only heparin. Other cells containing granules had been described and the peripheral blood basophil was believed to be similar to the mast cell because of the morphological appearance and the histochemical properties of the cytoplasmic granules. There is continued debate as to whether the basophil represents the circulating equivalent of the tissue mast cell, although there is insufficient evidence to support a close association. From the humble beginnings of a colourful cell containing a single chemical substance, the mast cell has grown in physiological importance and chemical complexity, as it is now known that numerous biologically active substances are produced by a single mast cell. The recognized mediators, heparin, histamine, proteases, prostaglandins and leukotrienes, are among the potent biologically active compounds. The granule contains preformed mast cell products while other mediators are actively synthesized after mast cell stimulation (Galli, 1987).

Complex mast cell physiology

The mast cell plays an important role in the normal immunological process and forms one of the critical elements in diseases related to immediate hypersensitivity. The presence of specific IgE class receptors on the mast cell surface provides one mechanism to explain specific antigen activation of mast cell degranulation. In addition to specific IgE mediated events, many physical events and chemical compounds cause mast cell degranulation which makes it attractive to think the mast cell has an important physiological role in non-immunological processes. The wide distribution of the mast cell in the various tissues of the body and the nature of its intracellular contents provides a convenient mechanism for the focal delivery of specific active compounds in response to a number of environmental stimuli. In addition to providing endogenous mast cell products, the mast cell concentrates exogenous substances within its cytoplasmic granules which can be released with mast cell activation. Despite these suggestive pathophysiologic links, it is difficult to confirm the role the mast cell plays in non-immunological physiology. A self-regulatory role for the mast cell is suggested by the evidence that mast cell activation induces mast cell proliferation (Galli, 1987). This self-regulatory role is particularly important in the gastrointestinal tract as this process can help explain a 'sensitization' process. In our patients with regional gastrointestinal mast cell related disease, we have observed that symptoms often begin with a discrete allergic-like reaction following a prolonged self-perpetuated course.

Difficulties in studying the physiological role of mast cells

One of the experimental difficulties in clarifying the role of the mast cell in a specific biological response is isolating the effects of mast cell degranulation from other simultaneous physiological events. Unfortunately, drugs used to alter mast cell function influence other biological processes, confusing the issue. Understanding the molecular biology of the mast cell is complicated further by the recent observation that there are numerous subgroups of mast cells (Befus et al., 1985). Each subgroup of mast cells stains differently due to the differences in their intracellular products. These differences have been supported by electron microscopic assessment of cellular ultrastructure. Heterogeneity of the gastrointestinal mast cells would be useful in explaining variable reactivity and sensitivity of patients to the different pathophysiological processes that degranulate mast cells. Variable intracellular composition permits different mast cell expression from an immunological and physiological point of view. The tissue microenvironment directly affects mast cell expression by influencing mast cell degranulation and the paracrine response to the products released. In addition, microenvironment influences subclass proliferation of specific mast cells. Mast cell heterogeneity and microenvironment adaptation allow patients to respond selectively to environmental stimuli by activating unique subclasses of mast cells.

Role of the mast cell in patients

It is unclear whether the important symptoms associated with disorders of mast cell function are related to specific IgE-mediated processes or the non-specific causes for mast cell degranulation. Non-immunological factors causing mast cell degranulation include many physical as well as chemical stimuli. It appears that non-immunological mast cell degranulation must occur if the symptom complex associated with mastocytosis represents mast cell degranulation, since these patients do not have sufficient documentation of IgE-mediated events. Of particular interest in gastroenterology are the mast cell degranulating substances found in food or food additives. Other degranulating factors include stress, heat, cold, insect bites, many drugs including aspirin, non-steroidal drugs as well as alcohol.

SYSTEMIC MASTOCYTOSIS

The clinical disorder 'mastocytosis' has traditionally been divided into cutaneous and systemic mastocytosis. In systemic mastocytosis, prominent organ involvement can occur in the liver, spleen and bone marrow. In addition, specific mast cell-related tumours have been identified in the stomach as well as the small intestine. It has been estimated that one out of every 8000 patients in a dermatology clinic (Lewis, 1984) has cutaneous mastocytosis. Formerly, the presence of skin lesions typical of cutaneous mastocytosis was essential for the diagnosis of systemic mastocytosis. Recently, Roberts *et al.* (1982) identified systemic mastocytosis without urticaria pigmentosa as a frequent cause of recurrent syncope. Since cutaneous mastocytosis represents focal increases in cutaneous mast cells without systemic involvement, it seems reasonable that other areas of the body (especially the gastrointestinal tract) may also exhibit symptomatic regional proliferation of mast cells. In several patients we have evaluated, we have found variable numbers of mast cells in different tissues. This suggests the 'systemic' mastocytosis, could probably be defined most accurately as patients with systemic symptoms and a documented increase in mast cells in one region, rather than the current implication that there is a diffuse increase in tissue mast cells.

Symptoms

Symptoms in systemic mastocytosis are so numerous and so difficult to explain that the physician unaware of the diagnosis often throws up his hands in frustration (Table 15.1). In patients with systemic mastocytosis much of the psychiatric disturbance is related to the frustration of a poorly understood complex of serious symptoms (Rogers *et al.*, 1986). The fact the patient does not believe that his physician understands the complexity of his numerous symptoms in relationship to the medical history causes depression. Table 15.2 illustrates the most common symptoms associated with mastocytosis in three different series. This data may reflect (a) the differences in reporting that exist related to the subspecialty perspective of the physicians, (b) the probability that the patient

Table 15.1. Symptoms in patients with systemic mastocytosis

Fatigue	Dizziness
Poor circulation	Nausea
Flushing	Vomiting
Headaches	Diarrhoea
Fainting	Faecal incontinence
Chest pain	Abdominal pain
Pruritis	Urinary frequency
Breathlessness	Muscle/joint pain
Hallucinations	Numbness/tingling
Palpitations	

Table 15.2. Comparison of major symptoms in different series of patients with systemic mastocytosis and IBS

Symptom	Systemic mastocytosis (%)			IBS (%)
	Sample 1 (*N* = 16)	Sample 2 (*N* = 21)	Sample 3 (*N* = 26)	Sample 4 (*N* = 100)
Abdominal pain	75	75	40	100
Diarrhoea	62	75	40	41
Headache	19	>50	20	34
Flushing	44	95	32	?
Pruritis	88	95	44	32
Palpitations	31	90	?	51
Joint and back pain	19	?	20	61

References: for sample 1, Cherner *et al.* (1988); for sample 2, Roberts *et al.* (1982); for sample 3, Webb *et al.* (1982); for sample 4, Whorwell *et al.* (1986).

may have different symptoms related to the different numbers of mast cells in different regions.

A large proportion of patients with systemic mastocytosis have cutaneous flushing associated with hypotension and occasionally frank shock. The flushing episodes must be distinguished from those of the carcinoid syndrome, which is the principle differential diagnostic consideration in patients with mastocytosis. The symptoms listed in Table 15.1 can be induced by a number of environmental stimuli including specific foods, alcohol, aspirin, heat, anxiety, stress, and physical exercise. The gastrointestinal symptoms in systemic mastocytosis are similar to the symptoms in the regional disorders of mast cell proliferation in the gastrointestinal tract and are discussed in detail below.

The reported association of malignancy in patients with systemic mastocytosis is difficult to verify. Mast cell proliferation occurs in *response* to neoplasm, but whether it precedes neoplastic disease is unknown. A true pathogenic association between malignancy and mastocytosis is difficult to believe, since mastocytosis in young people often disappears as they grow older.

Diagnosis

Diagnosing systemic mastocytosis is difficult. Strictly speaking, mastocytosis implies an increase in the number of mast cells due to hyperplasia or neoplasia. Mast cell neoplasia is rare but certainly does occur with either localized mastocytomas or mast cell leukaemia. Increased numbers of mast cells are easily identifiable in the skin lesions of urticaria pigmentosa, erythroderma mastocytosis, diffuse infiltrated mastocytosis and telangiectasia macularis eruptiva persitans. Although skin lesions help make the diagnosis of systemic mastocytosis, Roberts *et al.* (1982) have shown that systemic mastocytosis without urticaria pigmentosa is fairly frequent. They satisfied the requirement for documenting an increase in mast cell numbers by obtaining biopsies from apparently uninvolved skin of patients with syncope of unknown origin. The increased number of mast cells in these blind biopsies was useful in establishing the diagnosis. An increase in the number of mast cells is currently the histological gold standard to diagnose mastocytosis, although theoretically the symptoms of mastocytosis could occur if there were mast cells with overactive metabolic processes increasing the quantity of mast cell mediators or if the patient had delayed metabolism of mast cell products. Increased mast cells have been demonstrated in the bone marrow, lymph nodes, liver, spleen and small bowel of patients with systemic mastocytosis. In our experience, many patients with a typical presentation for systemic mastocytosis often do not have increased mast cells in all tissues biopsied. We have developed sufficient experience to identify increased numbers of mast cells in the mucosa of the stomach and colon of individuals with symptoms of mastocytosis. The observation that many of our patients with systemic symptoms often have normal numbers of mast cells in some of their biopsies has lead us to expand the concept of regional mast cell disease in the skin to a regional gastrointestinal mast cell disease.

Laboratory diagnosis

Since this active metabolic cell produces numerous chemical compounds, identification of one of them in blood, urine, or tissue ought to help establish a diagnosis of systemic mastocytosis. The most obvious candidate is histamine. Unfortunately, histamine has a very short half-life in the blood and the diagnosis by blood testing requires active mast cell degranulation. A false positive result can arise secondary to increased histamine from the tissue disrupted with the needle puncture. An elevated histamine level in the urine should accurately identify patients with systemic mastocytosis, since the mast cell is responsible for histamine production. Indeed, a 24-

hour urine collection with the measurements done by a reliable laboratory can be helpful in making this diagnosis. Identifying histamine in the urine is a difficult process as the release from mast cells must be markedly elevated to increase urinary values. In addition, decarboxylation of histidine by the bacteria in the female bladder or vagina can cause exogenous contamination of the urine and false elevation of the histamine concentrations. Measurement of the metabolic products of histamine, N-methyl histamine and N-methylimidazole acetic acid (Keyzer *et al.*, 1983), eliminates false negative results and avoids the false positive caused by bacteria by quantifying the metabolic products of histamine not produced by bacteria. This is useful in the hands of experts; however, these measurements are not available for the non-research-oriented clinician. Tissue histamine has been measured in skin and gastric tissue as an index of elevated mast cell numbers (Ammann *et al.*, 1976), although it is again difficult to obtain these values and standards are lacking with regard to the quantitative results as well as a uniform procedure for collecting the samples.

Since mast cell degranulation stimulates prostaglandin D_2 production, measurement (Roberts *et al.*, 1980) of the urinary metabolites of prostaglandin D_2 should reflect an increased number of activated mast cells. This is an extremely difficult test requiring mass spectrometry and the difficult monitoring of the internal standards. This is an impractical test at the present time.

A third potentially useful plasma or serum test is tryptase levels (Schwartz *et al.*, 1987). Tryptase is a highly selective marker for mast cells which can be detected hours after a precipitating event such as an attack of anaphylaxis. The prolonged elevation of tryptase is probably due to (a) a slower diffusion from the site of degranulated mast cells than with histamine, and (b) a longer half-life than histamine. Even though this is a potentially useful test for the diagnosis of mast cell degranulation, only 11 of the 16 patients with systemic mastocytosis studied by Schwartz *et al.* (1987) had tryptase levels above the hospital control population

These problems document the frustration of trying to establish a diagnosis of systemic mastocytosis by biochemical tests. A useful provocative test has not been established which can safely induce mast cell degranulation. A morphine stimulation test was advocated in the past; however, the potential of a life-threatening reaction makes this an improper way to diagnosis mastocytosis.

Two diseases must be excluded before making a diagnosis of systemic mastocytosis. The first is carcinoid syndrome, which can present with flushing and hypotension, and the second is phaeochromocytoma, which can present with flushing and hypertension. It is most important to eliminate the carcinoid syndrome by urinary 5-HIAA (hydroxyindole-acetic acid) measurement prior to diagnosing mastocytosis. Increased histamine in the urine has been noted in carcinoid syndrome although this certainly must be very rare (Oates & Sjoerdsma, 1962).

MAST CELLS AND THE GASTROINTESTINAL TRACT

There are several potential roles for the mast cell in the pathophysiology of gastrointestinal symptoms. First, there is the proper role of the mast cell as an integral part of the body's immunological defense; second, there is the effect of systemic mastocytosis on gastrointestinal pathophysiology and function; the third role is the identification of the mast cell in established gastrointestinal diseases; and fourth, there may be a regional proliferation of mast cells in the gastrointestinal tract with no other systemic or gastrointestinal disease to account for the increased mast cells.

Gastrointestinal symptoms in systemic mastocytosis

The numerous mediators released with mast cell degranulation have potent effects on gastrointestinal motility, secretion, perception of pain, inflammatory response and vascular supply. Histamine is the most prominent of these mast cell mediators; however, serotonin, exoglycodiasase, prostaglandin D_2, leukotrienes B_4 and C_5, prostaglandin generating factor and chemotactic factors for the eosinophil and neutrophil also mediate these potent, gastrointestinal events. With this biochemical potential, it is not surprising that patients with systemic mastocytosis have a variety of symptoms relevant to the gastrointestinal tract (Table 15.1). Nausea and vomiting occur in over one-half of the cases (Roberts *et al.*, 1982) and episodic diarrhoea occurs in one-fifth. In addition, there are a number of isolated reports suggesting that the well-known effect of histamine on gastric acid secretion causes symptomatic acid peptic disease. The casual observation that mild steatorrhoea and symptoms of gastric acid hypersecretion are common has not been subjected to prospective analysis until recently (Cherner *et al.*, 1988). Sixteen consecutive patients with systemic mastocytosis were prospectively evaluated for a number of gastrointestinal abnormalities. Thirteen had significant gastrointestinal symptoms.

Abdominal pain and diarrhoea were the most prominent symptoms. Nine patients had dyspeptic gastrointestinal symptoms which improved after treatment with H_2 antagonists. Six patients with non-dyspeptic pain symptoms did not respond to H_2 antagonist treatment. In our experience, many of these patients will respond to H_1 antagonists, suggesting the pain is not acid related. Endoscopic evaluation demonstrated visible mucosal disease in eight of the 16 patients; however, only three patients had duodenal ulcers.

Five other patients had severe or moderate inflammation in the duodenum.

Histological findings are not reported. Mast cells are difficult to demonstrate in gastrointestinal mucosa due to their staining properties. In our evaluation of over 500 mucosal biopsies for mast cells we determined that five mast cells per high power field is the mean, median and mode in intestinal mucosa. In patients with well documented systemic mastocytosis, the number of mast cells demonstrated by endoscopic biopsy can vary in the antrum, duodenum, colon and terminal ileum. There are patients with systemic mastocytosis who have increased mast cell numbers in skin and bone marrow but not in the gastrointestinal tract. The possible explanations for this observation are discussed later in the chapter.

Gastric analysis revealed a broad range of basal acid output. There was a significant relationship between plasma histamine levels and basal acid output; however, maximal acid secretion after pentagastrin (a reflection of parietal cell mass) was not correlated with plasma histamine concentration. Compared to normal subjects, serum gastrin levels were significantly lower in patients with systemic mastocytosis. The low serum gastrin levels provide important insight into the issue of gastric acid secretion. Gastrin is an important trophic factor for the parietal cells as high gastric levels increase the parietal cell mass. When histamine increases basal acid secretion, there is a compensatory acid-induced suppression of antral gastrin. The low (<20 pg/ml) fasting gastrin we have observed suggests that non-gastrin stimulated acid is weak support for the diagnosis of mastocytosis. Since the gastrin is low, it is not surprising that the parietal cell mass is normal and theoretically it may even be decreased, since histamine does not have a trophic effect on parietal cells. We have found low or moderate doses of H_2 (cimetidine 200–300 mg B.I.D.) antagonists effective in suppressing symptoms of acid-sensitive disease in most patients who are being treated with H_1 antagonists.

The second major symptom that has been reported in patients with mastocytosis is episodic diarrhoea. This occurred in about 70% of patients reported by Roberts *et al.* (1982) and in over 63% of the patients in Cherner's (1988) study. Cherner *et al.* (1988) observed that only half of the patients complaining of diarrhoea had faecal outputs greater than 200 g/day and 31% of the patients had evidence of mild malabsorption. The malabsorption appears to be due to diffuse small intestinal mucosal dysfunction, as fat, D-xylose and B_{12} absorption are all mildly abnormal. The granularity of the small bowel found in enteroclysis studies, and severe nodularity seen with conventional small bowel follow-through studies in patients with mastocytosis, reflect the anatomical changes associated with these findings. Despite the complaint of diarrhoea, only half the patients had increased faecal weight, suggesting that abnormal colonic and anorectal motility rather than intestinal secretion or steatorrhoea may account for this symptom.

Non-gastric histamine effects on the gastrointestinal tract include increasing secretion of fluid (McCabe & Smith, 1984), increasing intestinal myoelectric activity (Konturek & Siebers, 1980), and relaxing of the internal anal sphincter (Burleigh & D'Mello, 1983). Many patients with diarrhoea due to mastocytosis have severe rectal urgency and faecal incontinence. The anorectal studies in these patients reveal a number of abnormalities associated with relaxation of the internal anal sphincter, with and without balloon stimulation of the rectum. With these profound manometric changes, it is surprising that incontinence is not regularly mentioned as a prominent feature of gastrointestinal dysfunction in mastocytosis. Other gastrointestinal tests evaluated by Cherner *et al.* (1988) indicate that gastric emptying is slightly, but not significantly, more rapid in patients with mastocytosis and small bowel transit time was unchanged.

Increased gastrointestinal mucosal mast cells in known gastrointestinal diseases

Since the mast cells participate in the first line of immunological defense in the skin, nasal passages, lungs, and intestines, it is not surprising that they have been associated with a variety of gastrointestinal diseases. The obvious infectious disease in which mast cell numbers should be increased is parasitic infestation. This was the first important disease in which mast cells were correlated with gastrointestinal pathophysiology (Miller & Walshaw, 1972; Strobel *et al.*, 1981). With the complex immunology of inflammatory bowel disease, it might be expected that mast cells would be increased in Crohn's disease. Indeed, mast cell hyperplasia is present in inflammatory bowel disease (Ranlov *et al.*, 1972; Lloyd *et al.*, 1975). Recent work by Collins *et al.* suggests the mast cell may have an important role in the aetiology and symptoms of Crohn's disease (see Chapter 14). We have a large population of patients with inflammatory bowel disease who require repetitive colonoscopy and ileoscopy for evaluation of their disease. We have found several interesting findings in patients with inflammatory bowel disease. In most patients, there is a slight but unimpressive increase in the number of mast cells in mucosal biopsies, but there are occasional patients who have markedly increased mast cells throughout their bowel. The most notable findings occurred in patients with ulcerative colitis in complete remission being endoscoped for routine cancer surveillance. We are currently evaluating the number of mast cells in patients with active ulcerative colitis to determine the relationship of mast cells to active disease and effective therapy. Analysis of more specific colonic subclasses of disease may improve the discrimination of the biopsy results and allow more refined treatment.

Another obvious area for possible mast cell hyperplasia is immunological sensitization. Coeliac disease is the paradigm of gut sensitization as the immunological reaction to gluten has been carefully assessed. Increased numbers of mast cells are present in the small intestine biopsies in untreated coeliac disease and they return to normal after a gluten-free diet (Strobel *et al.*, 1983). When the stimulus (gluten) is removed, the improvement in histology corresponds with the decrease in the mast cell population. This increase and decrease in mast cell numbers with treatment is consistent with the self-regulatory aspect of mast cell function. Although the importance of the mast cell in coeliac disease is not known, the function of the mast cell in tissue injury and in attracting inflammatory cells is consistent with the pathophysiology of the disease.

Gastrointestinal mucosal mast cell heterogeneity

The issue of mast cell heterogeneity has complicated research pertaining to the human mucosal mast cells. Well delineated differences in the mast cells in different tissues requires us to re-evaluate the number and character of mast cells and to re-examine their function in the gastrointestinal tract. Evaluation of tissue fixatives and staining techniques suggests that routine histochemical techniques are inadequate to evaluate the gastrointestinal mucosal mast cells properly, and standards need to be established in each laboratory. We use a low pH (pH 0.5) alcian blue stain on endoscopic biopsy tissue fixed in formalin for documenting the number of mast cells. We have evaluated a number of fixatives including Carnoy's, Bouin's, and formalin. In contrast to Befus *et al.* (1985) and Ruitenberg *et al.* (1982), we did not find better mast cell counts using Carnoy's solution. Our failure to confirm these findings regarding the fixative emphasizes the need for standards to be developed in each clinical or research laboratory. We agree with Befus *et al.* (1985) that there are at least two morphological types of mast cells identifiable in the small intestine, suggesting variability in intracellular contents of different mast cells in the intestine. Evaluation of the mast cells with regard to symptoms and the factors which cause mast cell degranulation will be an important research area as our understanding of the nature and importance of these histochemical differences becomes clearer.

Regional mast cell disease

Mastocytosis has traditionally been divided into systemic or cutaneous mastocytosis. It is probably naive to assume that the only 'regional' mast cell disease is that of cutaneous mastocytosis. We have documented several patients with increased mast cell numbers in the gastrointestinal mucosa, and no change in mast cell numbers on skin or bone marrow biopsies. Many of the patients with high numbers of mucosal mast cells were referred for evaluation because they failed to have a diagnosis made using the usual investigative procedures or they did not respond to the drugs routinely used in clinical gastroenterology. In assessment of these patients, we biopsied the fundus of the stomach, the gastric antrum, the duodenum, the terminal ileum and numerous sites in the colon for gastrointestinal mucosal mast cells. Antral biopsies correlated best with clinical symptoms. Figure 15.1 illustrates the mast cell distribution in antral biopsies from 195 patients endoscoped for a variety of medical indications. The average number of mast cells was 5.2 per high power field with a standard error of 0.32. There were 21 patients with more than 10 mast cells per high power field. In these patients, the histological diagnosis, excluding evaluation of the specific stains for mast cells, was gastritis, while nine were normal. We observed that a mast cell count greater than 10 per high power field was consistently associated with symptoms of abdominal pain and nausea. Patients usually responded to treatment with high dose H_1 antagonists alone (chlorpheniramine, 32 mg/day), but we occasionally needed to add a low dose H_2 antagonist. When the antral biopsies in patients with recognized gastric diseases were evaluated, no disorder had a pattern of raised mast cell counts. For example, in the antral biopsies from 15 patients with *Helicobacter pylori*, the average mast cell count is 3.3 per high power field, with no biopsy having greater than 10 mast cells per high power field. We expect that patients with high numbers of mast cells in the antrum can be considered to have a 'regional' mast cell disorder.

In patients with well documented systemic mastocytosis on the basis of urticaria pigmentosa, positive bone marrow biopsies and systemic symptoms, gastrointestinal symptoms are usually present (Table 15.2). Interestingly, we do not always find increased mast cell numbers in biopsies of their gastrointestinal mucosa. The symptoms in patients with systemic mastocytosis without increased mucosal mast cell numbers are similar to symptoms in patients with regional gastrointestinal mast cell disease. This suggests mast cell degranulation has an endocrine effect in addition to the expected paracrine effect. There are several broad implications of these observations. (a) 'Systemic' mastocytosis may represent a disease in which the symptoms are systemic, but the mast cell proliferation is regional. In this instance, there may be an identifiable and remediable focal cause for the mast cell proliferation. (b) Sensitivity to the systemic effects of mast cell disease may vary among patients. This may be misleading with regard to diagnosis, as the patient

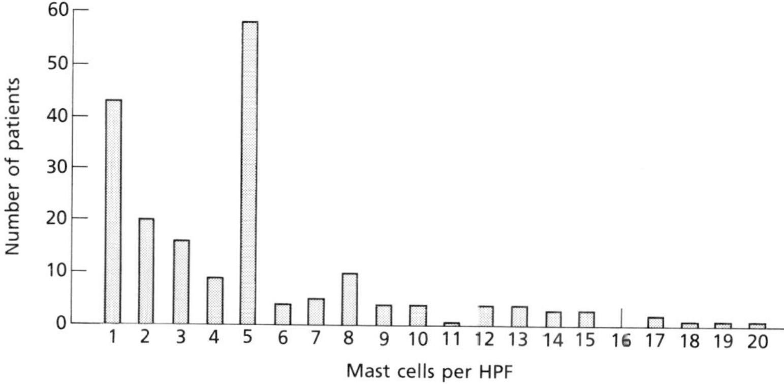

Fig. 15.1. Mast cell distribution in antral biopsies during endoscopy for various medical indications.

concentrates on seeking medical care for the prominent symptoms. For instance, the patient may complain of severe headaches and attribute the nausea and vomiting of gastrointestinal mastocytosis to the headache rather than attributing the headache to the gastrointestinal mast cell degranulation. (c) The symptoms of gastrointestinal mast cell disease include episodic diarrhoea and abdominal pain which may mimic other disorders such as irritable bowel syndrome (IBS). The gastrointestinal and systemic symptoms in patients with IBS reported by Whorwell *et al.* (1986—see Table 15.2) could be explained by the systemic effects of gastrointestinal mast cell degranulation. In an uncontrolled fashion, I have had a favourable clinical experience with H_1 antagonists in treating some patients with IBS and systemic symptoms.

Increased mast cells limited to the gut may be caused by sensitization to food or drink or a viral illness. This is consistent with the medical history related by patients with regional gastrointestinal mast cell disease, discussed above. Once initiated, the patient notices continued symptoms of increasing severity. Moneret-Vautrin *et al.* (1984) suggest that the change in permeability caused by mast cell degeneration and the self-proliferation of mast cells induced by degranulation accounts for this vicious cycle. The subclass of patients with an abrupt onset respond well to cromolyn therapy. Cromolyn is a poorly absorbed mast cell stabilizer although it does have a beneficial systemic effect in some patients with mastocytosis (Soter *et al.*, 1979). This suggests that controlling gastrointestinal mast cell numbers may decrease mast cell stimulation in the rest of the body. After 6–8 months of aggressive cromolyn treatment without recurrent systemic symptoms, several patients have been able to decrease their medications gradually without a recurrence of the symptoms. In some of these patients repeat biopsies show a marked fall in the number of mast cells. A hypothesis consistent with these findings would implicate an insult that would cause mast cell proliferation because of a specific antigen or non-specific mast cell stimulation. After the release of mast cell contents, an increase in intestinal permeability of the small bowel would allow further mast cell recruitment and provide an opportunity for continued stimulation to occur by other specific or non-specific substances. With the increase in the number of mast cells, a permanent change in gastrointestinal permeability would allow molecules of different sizes to continue mast cell stimulation. The permeability changes seen in Crohn's disease and coeliac disease are consistent with the suggestion of increased intestinal permeability. Abnormal numbers of mast cells in coeliac disease return to normal after a gluten-free diet (Strobel *et al.*, 1983), as do the number of mast cells in patients I have treated who go into 'remission'.

TREATMENT OF SYSTEMIC MASTOCYTOSIS AND REGIONAL GASTROINTESTINAL MAST CELL DISEASE

The treatment of systemic mastocytosis is potentially complex because of the number of products which are released by the mast cell. Figure 15.2 illustrates areas of possible intervention in mast cell-related disease. The first goal is to decrease the precipitating factors. Clearly, this has value in many patients since the precipitating factors may be easily identified and eliminated to allow the patients to have symptom-free intervals. For example, alcohol is a common precipitating factor which is easily eliminated. Red wine is effective in causing symptoms as (a) alcohol induces mast cell degranulation; (b) the high content of bisulphites degranulates mast cells; and (c) tyramine inhibits the metabolism of histamine by the gastrointestinal tract mucosa through competitive inhibition of the monoamine oxidase system.

Despite the complexity of mast cell degranulation and the number of mast cell mediators which are released, the use of H_1 antagonists is the most important aspect of managing patient symptoms, as they not only block the H_1 receptor but also seem to stabilize the mast cell. After mast cell stabilization, the release of non-histamine preformed products is decreased and there is blunting of stimulated synthesis of active mediators. If blocking the H_1 site is not sufficient or if dyspepsia continues despite H_1 blockade, a small dose of an H_2 antagonist (cimetidine, 300 mg daily) is often sufficient to manage the patient's symptoms. Blocking prostaglandin synthesis decreases another group of mast cell mediators. Aspirin is an obligatory degranulator of mast cells and treatment must be initiated with *extreme caution* to avoid a serious attack. In addition to blocking prostaglandin synthesis, aspirin may prevent serious attacks by causing continual low grade mast cell

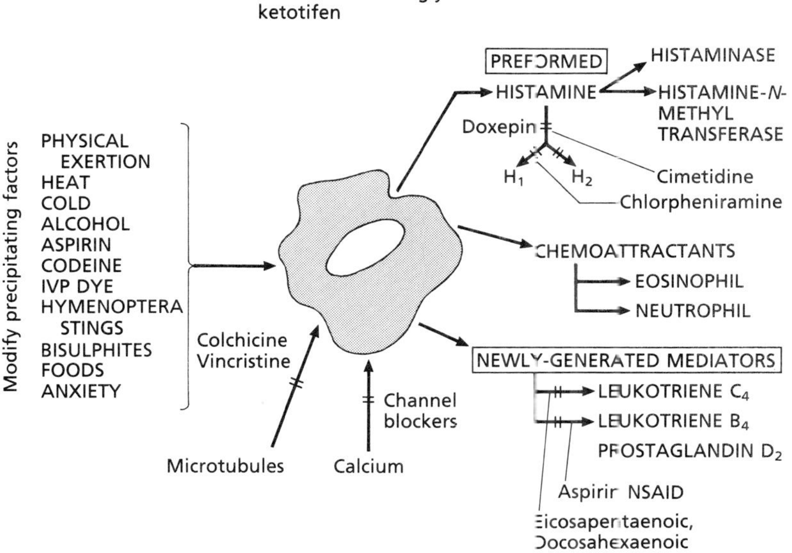

Fig. 15.2. Areas of possible intervention in mast cell-related disease.

degranulation and eliminating the burst potential of degranulation. Cromolyn is a mast cell stabilizer with an interesting effect in systemic disease. Even though it is not absorbed effectively by the gastrointestinal tract, it improves symptoms in a number of patients, particularly those with upper gastrointestinal symptoms. Doses as low as 100 mg/day have been effective in managing several regional gastrointestinal mast cell disease patients, although higher doses are recommended for systemic disease (Soter *et al.*, 1979). Ketotifen is a mast cell stabilizer with antihistamine effects. This is an important drug because it is readily absorbed from the gastro-intestinal tract and has proved to be very effective in the chronic urticaria syndrome. Management of patients with ketotifen holds great hope in the future with regard to systemic mastocytosis, and controlled trials are under way, assessing its efficacy. The other drugs which are illustrated in Fig. 15.1 have theoretical advantages, and case reports have indicated that calcium channel blockers and microtubular inhibitors may be important in managing the disease, but little objective evidence is present to justify the use of these drugs outside of limits imposed by controlled clinical trials.

SUMMARY

Gastrointestinal mucosal mast cells are becoming increasingly recognized as being important in the origin of disease and in rela-tion to gastrointestinal symptoms. Patients with systemic diseases involving the mast cell as well as regional mast cell-related diseases can have complex and severe gastrointestinal symptoms. Standards for quantifying mucosal mast cells are being established and biopsies should be used to try to identify the gastrointestinal mucosal mast cells. As we look at other diseases, particularly inflammatory bowel disease, we may find that the mast cell creates a paradigm for gastrointestinal symptoms and inflammation.

REFERENCES

Ammann, R.W., Veter D., Deyhle, P., Tschen, H., Sulser, H., & Schmid, M. (1976) Gastrointestinal involvement in systemic mastocytosis. *Gut* **17**, 107–112.

Befus, D., Goodacre, R., Dyck, N. & Bienenstock, J. (1985) Mast cell heterogeneity in man: I. Histologic studies of the intestine. *Int Arch Allergy Appl Immun* **76**, 232–236.

Burleigh, D.E. & D'Mello, A. (1983) Neural and pharmacologic factors affecting motility of the internal anal sphincter. *Gastroenterology* **84**, 409–417.

Cherner, J.A., Jensen, R.T., Dubois, A., O'Dorisio, T.M., Gardner, J.D. & Metcalfe, D.D. (1988) Gastrointestinal dysfunction in systemic mastocytosis: a prospective study. *Gastroenterology* **95**, 659–667.

Galli, S.J. (1987) New approaches for the analysis of mast cell maturation, heterogeneity, and function. Federation Proceedings **76**, 1906–1914.

Keyzer, J.J., Demonchy, J.G.R., Van Doormaal, J.J. & Van Voorst Vader, P.C. (1983) Improved diagnosis of mastocytosis by measurement of urinary histamine metabolites. *N Engl J Med* **309**, 1603–1605.

Konturek, S.J. & Siebers, R. (1980) Role of histamine H_1 and H_2 receptors on myoelectric activity of small bowel in the dog. *Am J Physiol* **238**, G50–56.

Lewis, R.A. (1984) Mastocytosis. *J Allergy Clin Immunol* **74**, 755–765.

Lloyd, G., Green, F.H.Y., Fox, H., Mani, V. & Turnberg, L.A. (1975) Mast cells and immunoglobulin E in inflammatory bowel disease. *Gut* **16**, 861–866.

McCabe, R.D. & Smith, P.L. (1984) Effects of histamine and histamine receptor antagonists on ion transport in rabbit descending colon. *Am J Physiol* **247**, G411–G418.

Miller, H.R.P. & Walshaw, R. (1972) Immune reactions in mucous membranes: histochemistry of intestinal mast cells during helminth expulsion in the rat. *Pathology* **69**, 195–206.

Moneret-Vautrin, D.A., Dekorwin, J.D., Tisserant, J., Grignon, M. & Claudot, N. (1984) Ultrastructural study of the mast cells of the human duodenal mucosa. *Clin Rev Allergy* **14**, 471–481.

Oates, J.A. & Sjoerdsma, A. (1962) A unique syndrome associated with secretion of 5-hydroxytryptophan by metastatic gastric carcinoids. *Am J Med* **32**, 333–342.

Ranlov, P., Nielsen, M.H. & Waustrupt, J. (1972) Ultrastructure of the ileum in Crohn's disease: immune lesions and mastocytosis. *Scand J Gastroenterol* **7**, 471–476.

Roberts, L.J., Sweetman, B.J., Lewis, R.A., Austen, K.F. & Oates, J.A. (1980) Increased production of prostaglandin D_2 in patients with systemic mastocytosis. *N Engl J Med* **303**, 1400–1404.

Roberts, L.J., Fields, J.P. & Oates, J.A. (1982) Mastocytosis without urticaria pigmentosa: a frequently unrecognized cause of recurrent syncope. *Trans Assoc Am Phys* **95**, 36–41.

Rogers, M.P., Bloomingdale, K., Murawski, B.J., Soter, N.A., Reich, P. & Avsten, K.F. (1986) Mixed organic brain syndrome as a manifestation of systemic mastocytosis. *Psychosom Med* **48**, 437–447.

Ruitenberg, E.J., Gustowska, L., Elgersma, A. & Ruitenberg, H.M. (1982) Effect of fixation on the light microscopical visualization of mast cells in the mucosa and connective tissue of the human duodenum. *Int Arch Allergy Appl Immun* **67**, 233–238.

Schwartz, L.B., Metcalfe, D.D., Miller J.S., Earl, H. & Sullivan, T. (1987) Tryptase levels as an indicator of mast cell activation in systemic anaphylaxis and mastocytosis. *N Engl J Med* **316**, 1622–1626.

Soter, N.A., Austen, K.F. & Wasserman, S.I. (1979) Oral disodium cromoglycate in the treatment of systemic mastocytosis. *N Engl J Med* **301**, 465–469.

Strobel, S., Miller, H.R.P., Ferguson, A. (1981) Human intestinal mucosal mast cells: evaluation of fixation and staining techniques. *J Clin Path* **34**, 851–858.

Strobel, S., Busuttil, A. & Ferguson, A. (1983) Human intestinal mucosal mast cells: expanded population in untreated coeliac disease. *Gut* **24**, 222–227.

Webb, T.A., Li, C.Y. & Yam, L.T. (1982) Systemic mast cell disease: a clinical and haematopathologic study of 26 cases. *Cancer* **49**, 927–938.

Whorwell, P.J., McCallum, M., Creed, F.H. & Roberts, C.T. (1986) Non-colonic features of irritable bowel syndrome. *Gut* **27**, 37–40.

16 *Lessons from Asthma*

P.H. Howarth

INTRODUCTION

Asthma is a disorder of the conducting airways characterized by obstruction to airflow which varies with time either spontaneously or in response to treatment. A number of mechanisms contribute to the airflow obstruction, including smooth muscle constriction, oedema and cellular infiltration of the airway wall and lumenal obliteration by inspissated mucus and cellular debris, in particular shed epithelial cells. The relative importance of each of these mechanisms will vary both between individuals and within an individual, depending upon both the disease activity and the provoking stimulus. It is, however, the recent recognition of the underlying importance of the cellular infiltration of the airways, and the realization that asthma is an inflammatory disease, that has permitted a major advance in the understanding of this disease. Prior to this, asthma was considered a disorder of smooth muscle and considerable research emphasis was directed towards the understanding of the neuromuscular control of airway calibre. It is this historical perspective which will be presented in this chapter, culminating in the present understanding of the complex neurocellular interactions in asthma and how an understanding of the mechanisms in this respiratory disorder could be of potential relevance to gastrointestinal disorders such as the irritable bowel.

BRONCHIAL HYPERRESPONSIVENESS

In 1921, Alexander and Padock observed 'asthmatic breathing' in asthmatic but not normal subjects following subcutaneous injections of pilocarpine. Because epinephrine promptly relieved the attacks, these investigators inferred that the symptoms were due to bronchoconstriction, and they speculated that the basic abnormality in asthma was an imbalance between the cholinergic and sympathetic nervous control of smooth muscle. Weiss *et al.* (1932), while investigating the systemic effects of intravenous histamine, discovered that small amounts of histamine precipitated attacks of bronchospasm and a decrease in vital capacity in subjects 'prone to bronchial asthma'. They subsequently showed that this response did not occur in normal subjects, despite doses of histamine that produced circulatory changes. Their initial observations were extended and confirmed over the next 20 years with respect to cholinergic drugs as well as histamine. Subsequently this enhanced responsiveness of the bronchi in asthma was demonstrated to occur to a wide variety of physical, chemical and pharmacological stimuli, including serotonin, bradykinin, SRS-A (slow reacting substance of anaphylaxis) and its individual leukotriene components, prostaglandin $F_{2\alpha}$, prostaglandin D_2, platelet activating factor, adenosine, β-adrenoceptor antagonists, exercise, cold air, sulphur dioxide, 'fog', cigarette smoke and citric acid (Boushey *et al.*, 1980; Hardy *et al.*, 1984; Holgate *et al.*, 1987). As this enhanced bronchoconstrictor response in asthma is not receptor specific and occurs to a wide variety of stimuli, it has been termed 'non-specific bronchial hyperresponsiveness'.

While bronchial hyperresponsiveness is a usual feature of symptomatic asthma, and it has been proposed by the American Thoracic Society that evidence of bronchial hyperresponsiveness is mandatory for the diagnosis of asthma (Harris *et al.*, 1962), bronchial hyperresponsiveness and asthma are not synonymous. Bronchial hyperresponsiveness has been described in other conditions with airflow limitation, such as chronic obstructive airways disease, sarcoidosis and cystic fibrosis, in allied disorders such as rhinitis, in first degree relatives of asthmatics and in individuals with no respiratory symptoms identified during epidemiological studies (Boushey *et al.*, 1980; Lee *et al.*, 1983). In some instances this may reflect symptomatically unrecognized asthma, but in those patients with airflow limitation geometric factors are of importance. In airflow limitation related to smoking there is a close linear correlation between the decline in FEV_1 (forced expiratory volume) and the increase in methacholine responsiveness. Geometric factors, however, cannot account for bronchial hyperresponsiveness in asthma (Cartier *et al.*, 1982), and several hypotheses have been proposed relating to a neuronal imbalance, including β-adrenergic dysfunction, α-adrenergic excess, enhanced cholinergic expression and, more recently, a disturbance of the non-adrenergic, noncholinergic, peptidergic nervous system (Lee *et al.*, 1983; Barnes, 1988).

NEURAL MECHANISMS

Three neural innervations are pertinent to the airways, the parasympathetic (cholinergic) and sympathetic (adrenergic) components of the autonomic nervous system and the non-adrenergic, noncholinergic (NANC) system which has a peptidergic transmission.

While smooth muscle has a dense cholinergic supply (constrictor), it has no significant adrenergic innervation (Sheppard *et al.*, 1983), despite possessing large numbers of β-adrenoceptors (relaxant) and few α-adrenoceptors (constrictor). The autonomic airway tone is determined by the balance between the vagal efferent activity and circulating catecholamine (adrenaline) levels. The NANC nervous system, which has been well documented within the gastrointestinal tract as a modulator of smooth muscle function (Crema *et al.*, 1968; Burnstock 1972; Burnstock & Costa, 1973), has only recently been described within the human airways (Polak & Bloom, 1982) and is peptidergic in transmission. Evidence *in vitro* indicates that the NANC system has both inhibitory and excitatory properties. The inhibitory properties are likely to be mediated by vasoactive intestinal polypeptide (VIP), peptide histidine isoleucine (PHI) and polypeptide histidine methionine (PHM). These peptides have an identical distribution within the airways and are coded for within the same gene complex. They are potent relaxants of vascular and airway smooth muscle *in vitro* and, in addition, VIP may exert regulatory control over mast cell degranulation and secretion of water and mucus within the airways, thereby regulating mucociliary transport. VIP-immunoreactive nerves are often distributed with cholinergic nerves, and ultrastructural studies indicate that VIP may coexist in the same nerve terminals as acetylcholine. Thus, by being cotransmitted with acetylcholine, VIP may act as a neuromodulator. The excitatory properties of the NANC neural system are likely to be transmitted by substance P (SP) and the tachykinins, neurokinin A (NKA), neurokinin B (NKB), neuropeptide K (NPK) and eledoisin-like peptide as well as by calcitonin gene-related peptide (CGRP). Substance P and CGRP are both potent constrictors of airway smooth muscle.

The first neural theory to explain the underlying bronchoconstriction in asthma was that of β-adrenergic dysfunction, permitting unopposed α-adrenoceptor and cholinergic stimulation (Szentivanyi, 1968). While initially attractive and supported by evidence from extrapulmonary tissue, this could not be substantiated in asthma as there does not appear to be any β-adrenoceptor blockade or down-regulation in asthmatic airways. β-agonists are widely and successfully used in the treatment of asthmatic symptoms and no difference exists in the dose–response curves to inhaled β-agonists in asthmatic and non-asthmatic subjects (Tattersfield, 1982). The theory of excess α-adrenoceptor activity (Kneussl & Richardson, 1978) could not be fully explored until the advent of the specific α-antagonist, prazocin. As prazocin neither produces bronchodilatation nor inhibits histamine-induced bronchoconstriction, an abnormality of α-adrenoceptors in asthma is unlikely. A third proposal, that of increased cholinergic tone (Nadel, 1977), has more substance. While this undoubtedly occurs in some instances, it is considered now to be a secondary event related to epithelial disruption rather than an intrinsic abnormality in asthma. Consistent with this is the transient enhancement of bronchial responsiveness to inhaled histamine following exposure to stimuli which disrupt the airway epithelium, such as viral upper respiratory tract infections, nitrous oxide and ozone. With epithelial disruption, inhaled substances such as citric acid, histamine, prostaglandin $F_{2\alpha}$ and sulphur dioxide, whose bronchoconstrictor effects are inhibited by atropine pretreatment, are considered to stimulate airway irritant receptors leading to enhanced vagal efferent activity and thus airway smooth muscle constriction. The reflex nature of this response has been confirmed in animal studies. In addition, the loss of epithelial-derived antibronchoconstrictor agents will potentiate the vagal response and the corelease of neuropeptides may perpetuate the airway damage. An imbalance in the NANC neural system is now proposed as a factor in asthma development (Barnes, 1988), as the excitatory peptides, SP and CGRP, in addition to contracting airway smooth muscle, are pro-inflammatory. Substance P promotes microvascular leakage, stimulates mucus secretion, is chemokinetic for eosinophils and neutrophils and is known to degranulate mast cells. CGRP is a vasodilator and in conjunction with SP will promote tissue oedema, a characteristic histopathological finding in asthma. In view of these pro-inflammatory actions, it is also possible that an imbalance in the NANC nervous system could alter the behaviour of airway smooth muscle, as the enhanced bronchial responsiveness in asthma occurs at a myogenic level and is related to the neurohumoral environment, since asthmatic and non-asthmatic airway smooth muscle preparations do not differ *in vitro* in their responsiveness to constrictor agents such as histamine, prostaglandins and leukotrienes (Dahlen, 1983). To understand the local airway environment in asthma it is necessary to recognize the histopathology of asthma and the implications this has to the pathogenesis of the disease.

AIRWAY HISTOPATHOLOGY

A number of studies (Earle, 1953; Houston *et al.*, 1953; Dunnil, 1960), following the first description by Leyden (1886), have characterized the light microscopic histopathological features of fatal asthma as:

1 Obstruction of the lumen of the small airways with inspissated mucus, cellular debris and inflammatory cells.

2 Desquamation of the bronchial epithelium down to the level of the lamina propria with detachment of the superficial columnar cells.

3 Mucosal oedema.

4 Cellular infiltration of the airway walls with eosinophils, but also to a lesser extent lymphocytes and mononuclear cells.

5 An apparent thickening of the basement membrane.
6 Hypertrophy and hyperplasia of airways smooth muscle.

The relevance of these findings to the spectrum of asthma encountered in clinical practice is, however, uncertain, because fatal asthma represents one extreme and patients have often received intensive treatment, the histopathological influence of which is undefined.

A few studies have attempted to answer these points by obtaining bronchial biopsies *in vivo* under general anaesthesia for histopathological analysis. The results are conflicting. In a comparison of the light microscopic findings in bronchial biopsies from patients with asthma and chronic bronchitis, Glynn and Michaels (1960) found eosinophil and plasma cell infiltration of the lamina propria to be features of asthma, while epithelial cell loss, basement membrane thickening and smooth muscle hypertrophy were not consistent findings. In a later study, Salvato (1968) confirmed the tissue eosinophilia and emphasized the thickened hyalinized basement membrane as a characteristic of asthma. He also commented on a reduction in granulated mast cells during acute exacerbations, implicating the involvement of these cells. More recently, Cutz *et al.* (1978) described the ultrastructural features of the airways in two asthmatic children undergoing open lung biopsy during clinical remission, and compared these findings with those from two children who had died in status asthmaticus. The post-mortem changes of mucus plugging, goblet cell hyperplasia, 'basement membrane thickening', peribronchial smooth muscle hypertrophy and eosinophilic infiltration were identified in the asymptomatic asthmatics, suggesting that these changes are due to the disease process and are not treatment-related changes. Transmission electron microscopy showed that the mucus plugs consisted of moderately electron dense material containing degenerate epithelial cells and macrophages, and that the lumenal surfaces of the ciliated epithelial cells showed cytoplasmic blebs and abnormal cilia. The mucus plugging was most marked in those areas in which the cilia were most abnormal, suggesting that mucus plugging may be a consequence of cilial dysfunction. Electron microscopy also revealed that the subepithelial layer, commonly referred to as a 'thickened basement membrane', consisted of a plexiform arrangement of collagen fibrils under the basement membrane, separated from it by a thin layer of ground substance. These findings were comparable in the four asthmatic children studied. The only difference identified between those with asymptomatic asthma and those who died during an asthma attack was the greater number of peribronchial eosinophils and the degree of focal denudation of the mucosa. No physiological correlates were reported in this study, and indeed the numbers studied by biopsy *in vivo* ($n = 2$) would not have permitted any meaningful statistical analysis.

FIBREOPTIC BRONCHOSCOPY AND ASTHMA

The advent of flexible fibreoptic bronchoscopy has facilitated the investigation of the airways. This technique has, however, only recently been applied to asthma in view of concerns over its safety in this condition. If safety guidelines are adhered to, significant bronchoconstriction associated with the technique is prevented. Bronchoscopy enables direct vision of the airways, the sampling of lumenal cells by bronchoalveolar lavage for characterization and functional studies, and the attainment of endobronchial biopsies to investigate tissue cellular and neural events.

BRONCHOALVEOLAR LAVAGE

Fibreoptic bronchoscopy under local anaesthesia with bronchoalveolar lavage (BAL) has been used to obtain airway lumenal cells for both differential counts and functional studies. In asthma there is increased recovery of eosinophils and mast cells (Flint *et al.*, 1985; Godard *et al.*, 1987). The recovered mast cells have an increased spontaneous release of histamine *in vitro*, which correlates significantly with the resting level of non-specific bronchial responsiveness (Flint *et al.*, 1985). Bronchoalveolar lavage has also been performed before and after bronchial provocation in asthma to relate any cellular change to the development of bronchoconstriction or change in non-specific bronchial responsiveness.

Bronchial provocation with both allergens and occupational chemicals have been studied. With these bronchoprovocants, there is an increase in non-specific bronchial responsiveness in those subjects experiencing a dual asthmatic response (immediate bronchoconstriction followed by recovery, and subsequent late bronchoconstriction at 6–12 hours post-challenge) but not in those subjects experiencing a single response (immediate bronchoconstriction only). Thus, by selecting dual and single responders, attempts have been made to identify the cellular changes relevant to late bronchoconstriction and the associated changes in bronchial responsiveness. The immediate response is associated with mast cell degranulation and the local release of mediators, producing initially mucosal pallor and then erythema and oedema plus bronchoconstriction. The late asthmatic response is associated with increased recovery of eosinophils in BAL fluid following allergen (De Monchy *et al.*, 1985) and occupational (red cedar) exposure (Lam *et al.*, 1987) and an excess of neutrophils following toluene diisocyanate (TDI) challenge (Fabbri *et al.*, 1987). These findings suggest that acute inflammation of the airways is of relevance to the development of the late asthmatic bronchoconstrictor response. Further support for the involvement of inflammatory cells is derived from bronchoscopic studies of local allergen challenge of subsegmental bronchi in selected asthmatics who are known to be dual responders (Metzger *et al.*, 1987). In these subjects, lavage 48 hours post-challenge reveals an increased recovery of macrophages, eosinophils, neutrophils and T helper (CD4) lymphocytes. Changes in lymphocytes in BAL have also been described at 6 hours following inhalation allergen challenge, with increases in T suppressor (CD8) cells and falls in T helper (CD4) cells in single responders (Gonzalez *et al.*, 1987). The number of T helper cells (CD4) recovered was found to be significantly lower in single responders than in dual responders at the same time points. As a consequence it has been suggested (since T suppressor cells produce histamine-induced suppressor factor, which inhibits lymphocyte proliferation and lymphokine production) that these cells might control the inflammatory events within the airways following allergen challenge by preventing the release of mediators from T helper cells. An inability to recruit T suppressor (CD8) cells leads to a perpetuation of disease activity. Consistent with this, in the minority of asthmatics who are 'corticosteroid resistant', there is a decrease in the number and function of circulating T suppressor (CD8) lymphocytes.

There is some difficulty, however, in interpreting these cellular changes in BAL, as the exact site from which the lavage fluid is derived is uncertain and the volume of lavage fluid recovered often varies between patients and centres, making total cell counts of little value. More importantly, the relevance of lavage findings to tissue cellular events is undefined.

BRONCHIAL BIOPSIES

The majority of flexible fibreoptic bronchoscopic investigations in asthma have concentrated on airway lavages, but few have systematically analysed airway biopsy specimens. In an attempt to rectify this we have undertaken fibreoptic bronchoscopy in asthma under local anaesthesia in Southampton to obtain airway tissue and lavage samples. In eight clinically mild asthmatics, with FEV_1 values ranging from 70% to 130% predicted and with a range of moderate to mild airway non-specific responsiveness, the airway findings were compared to those in non-atopic non-asthmatic subjects. In the asthmatics there was a greater recovery of epithelial cells in the lavage fluid and a negative correlation existed between the bronchoalveolar lavage epithelial cell count and the level of non-specific bronchial responsiveness ($\rho = 0.64$; $P = 0.03$). In the lavage fluid the epithelial cells were in clumps, had intact intercellular junctions and appeared to have normal cilia, suggesting that there may be abnormal adherence between the epithelium and the basement membrane. Paradoxically, evidence for a difference in epithelial disruption between the two groups was less easy to define

in the biopsies, because mechanical distortion, due to the pinching
action of the forceps, led to artefactual epithelial disruption, thus
preventing a satisfactory analysis of any difference between asthmatic and non-asthmatic subjects.

Due to the mild spectrum of asthma studied no other differences
in the lavage cell counts were identified in these two groups. However, differences were apparent within the tissue specimens. In
the non-asthmatic subjects there was a thin basement membrane
beneath the epithelium, and the lamina propria and submucosa
contained few inflammatory cells and only a fine supporting structure of collagen. In contrast in the asthmatics, there was evidence of
inflammatory cell infiltration with eosinophils and lymphocytes.
The basement membrane region was thickened and ultrastructural
analysis identified a normal basement membrane with a thickened
layer of sub-basement membrane matrix which immunohisto-
chemically was composed of types 3 and 5 collagen and fibronectin,
suggesting a fibroblast origin. Stimulation of fibroblast activity
could be related to mast cell degranulation, since transmission
electron microscopy identified evidence of mast cell degranulation
in the asthmatics, a feature not identified in the non-asthmatic
subjects. There was also evidence of eosinophil accumulation within
post-capillary vessels and in the lamina propria of the asthmatic
airways, with electron microscopic evidence of eosinophil activation, as indicated by the reversal of the electron-dense major
basic protein central core.

The extent of the changes identified within these asthmatic airways was surprising in view of the apparently mild clinical spectrum
of their disease. This information from mild asthmatic subjects
does, however, support the findings in post-mortem specimens from
patients dying from acute severe asthma, and further strengthens
the evidence identifying asthma as an inflammatory disease.

NEUROCELLULAR INTERACTIONS

Following the initial consideration of asthma as a disorder of
airway neuromuscular control, it is apparent from the foregoing
account that there is increasing evidence to classify asthma as
an inflammatory disease and to link the airway inflammation
with abnormal physiology. In asthma significant correlations exist
between the bronchoalveolar lavage eosinophil, lymphocyte and
mast cell numbers and the level of non-specific bronchial responsiveness. In the experimental situation, allergen inhalation challenge
in atopic asthma induces changes in bronchial responsiveness
in subjects experiencing a dual (early and late) but not a single
(isolated early) response. Bronchoalveolar lavage at the time of
the late response, when the airway responsiveness is increasing,
identifies an influx of lymphocytes, eosinophils and monocytes.

Biopsy specimens reveal eosinophils palisading beneath the basement membrane in allergic asthma.

For these cells to arrive within the airways in an activated state, there have to be local factors promoting (a) the expression of cell surface receptors on circulating cells so that they attach to the vascular endothelial surface; (b) diapedesis through the vascular endothelium; (c) chemotaxis to the airway site; and (d) local activation. Until recently it was considered that the mast cell orchestrated these events in allergic asthma, since the mast cell, in having high affinity high density IgE receptors, is primed in the atopic state to interact with allergen and is appropriately placed within the airway tissue (Holgate *et al.*, 1986). The mast cell comprises 0.04–0.1% of the total activated cell population recovered with bronchoalveolar lavage in normal subjects, and there is a 3–5-fold increase in this population in allergic asthma (Agius *et al.*, 1987). However, it is now apparent that while the mast cell is central to the immediate airway response to allergen (Howarth *et al.*, 1978), the immediate response alone is not associated with changes in bronchial responsiveness, and that salbutamol, a potent inhibitor of immunologically stimulated airway mast cell degranulation, while abolishing the immediate airway response to allergen (Howarth *et al.*, 1978), has no influence on the development of the late asthmatic response to allergen challenge or the changes in bronchial responsiveness associated with this (Cockcroft & Murduck, 1987). This evidence would suggest that cells other than the mast cell orchestrate the late inflammatory airway events and the changes in bronchial responsiveness following allergen challenge. Further indirect support for the non-involvement of the mast cell in orchestrating airway inflammation and bronchial responsiveness in asthma is derived from challenge studies in asthma with the purine nucleotide, adenosine, or the adenine nucleotides adenosine monophosphate (AMP) and adenosine 5′-diphosphate (ADP). As both AMP and ADP are rapidly dephosphorylated to yield adenosine, their airway effects are likely to be mediated by adenosine. Inhalation of adenosine in asthma produces a concentration-dependent bronchoconstriction which is receptor specific, as the purine guanosine has no airway effects over a similar concentration range. The airway effects of adenosine are considered to be secondary to activation of mast cells, with release of histamine. Such an action has been shown *in vitro* with rat peritoneal mast cells and *in vivo*. The H_1-receptor antagonists terfenadine and astemizole have been shown to inhibit AMP-induced bronchoconstriction. Inhalation of AMP in atopic asthmatics produces immediate bronchoconstriction, but no late asthmatic response or alteration in non-specific bronchial responsiveness, indirectly indicating that the release of preformed mast cell mediators does not contribute to the airway events associated with hyperresponsiveness. The emphasis in asthma has now

moved away from the mast cell with the realization that cell types
other than mast cells and basophils possess IgE receptors (Capron
et al., 1987). The lymphocyte, the macrophage, the eosinophil and
the platelet have all been found to possess low affinity Fc receptors
(Fc_{II}) for IgE. Thus, allergen exposure may activate these cell types,
in addition to mast cells, and the local release of mediators and
cytokines from the other cell types following allergen exposure
is likely to modulate inflammatory cell infiltration and activation
within the airways. In attempting to dissect out mechanisms, allergen is used as a model, but it is likely that activation of cells such as
macrophages or lymphocytes by factors other than allergen could
initiate a similar process leading to non-allergic asthma.

The causal relationship between airway inflammation and
bronchial responsiveness is at present still speculative. However,
immunocytochemical staining techniques identify the presence
of the eosinophil-derived major basic protein (MBP) in sputum
and lavage samples of asthmatics and eosinophil derived cationic
protein (ECP) is also present within airway biopsy samples. Both
MBP and ECP can induce cilial abnormalities and epithelial disruption *in vitro* (Gleich *et al.*, 1984), and could account for the
increased epithelial shedding identified in our bronchoscopy study
and the epithelial disruption and cilial abnormalities described in
mild asthma from rigid bronchoscopic studies in asthma. Epithelial
damage will expose afferent neural endings to stimulation by
inflammatory mediators and inhaled agents, leading to reflex neural
activity. Release of SP, tachykinins and CGRP by the NANC neural
system would result in bronchoconstriction, mucus hypersecretion,
microvascular leakage and vasodilatation, the latter two promoting
mucosal oedema and plasma exudation, all features apparent in
clinical asthma. This process would be opposed by the local release
of VIP following reflex cholinergic transmission. VIP is a relaxant
of airways smooth muscle and a regulator of mast cell, water and
mucus secretion within the airways. An imbalance between the
excretory and inhibitory properties of the NANC neural system as a
consequence of inflammation could, therefore, lead to the development of symptoms characteristic of the asthmatic state.

CONCLUSION

It has been possible to advance the understanding of the pathogenesis of bronchial challenge in asthma, through measurement of
the physiological airway response and the dissection of the processes involved in this, by the measurement of circulatory and local
mediator changes as indicators of cell activation, the identification
of cellular changes in both lavage and tissue sites, the application of
immunocytochemistry to differentiate cell populations, and from
an understanding of the mechanisms whereby cellular and neural

events can lead to symptom expression. Such an approach, although not so straightforward, would be applicable to irritable bowel disease. Indeed such an approach has been utilized, using balloon distension of the rectosigmoid and rectum to mimic the arrival of stool (Whitehead *et al.*, 1980). Thus a physiological model exists which could be applied, in a similar fashion as with the investigation of asthma, to dissect out mechanisms in irritable bowel disease. It is apparent from studies in asthma that the purine nucleotide, adenosine, can induce rapid smooth muscle constriction secondary to degranulation of mast cells and the release of the preformed mediator histamine. In asthma there is evidence of purinergic–cellular interaction which may be of relevance to the gut. The identification of the importance of inflammation in asthma, however, would not be consistent with the concept that irritable bowel disease represents 'asthma of the bowel'. The changes in asthma of epithelial disruption, eosinophilic infiltration of the tissue and the excess deposition of sub-basement membrane collagen (types 3 and 5) would correspond closely with the recently described collagenous colitis rather than irritable bowel disease. Despite this, investigations into the underlying basis of asthma provide information concerning mechanisms regulating lumenal secretions, and regulation of smooth muscle function, which may have pertinence to other organs and provide a directional approach to the investigation of disordered function, as with irritable bowel disease.

REFERENCES

Agius, R.M., Howarth, P.H., Robinson, C. & Holgate, S.T. (1986) Human broncho-alveolar mast cells and their mediators. In Kay, A.B. (ed), *Asthma: Clinical Pharmacology and Therapeutic Progress*, pp. 274–285. BSP, Oxford.

Alexander, H.L. & Padock, R. (1921) Bronchial asthma: response to pilocarpine and epinephrine. *Arch Int Med* 27, 184–189.

Barnes, P.J. (1988) Airway neuropeptides. In Barnes, P.J., Rodger, I.W., Thompson, N.C. (eds), *Asthma: Basic Mechanisms and Clinical Management*, pp. 395–413. Academic Press, London.

Boushey, H.A., Holtzman, J., Sheller, J.R. & Nadel, J.A. (1980) Bronchial hyper-reactivity. *Am Rev Resp Dis* 121, 389–413.

Burnstock, G. (1972) Purinergic nerves. *Pharm Rev* 24, 509–581.

Burnstock, G. & Costa, M. (1973) Inhibitory innervation of the gut. *Gastroenterology* 64, 141–144.

Capron, A., Dessaint, J.-P. & Tonnel, A.B. (1987) IgE receptors on inflammatory cells. In Michel, F.B., Bousquet, J., Godard, P. (eds), *Highlights in Asthmology*, pp. 107–116. Springer-Verlag, Berlin.

Cartier, A., Thompson, N.C., Frith, P.A., Roberts, R. & Hargreave, F.E. (1982) Allergen-induced increase in bronchial responsiveness to histamine: relationship to the late asthmatic response and change in airway calibre. *J Allergy Clin Immunol* 70, 170–177.

Cockcroft, D.W. & Murdock, K.Y. (1987) Comparative effects of inhaled salbutamol, sodium cromoglycate, and beclomethasone dipropionate on allergen-induced early asthmatic responses, late asthmatic responses, and increased bronchial responsiveness to histamine. *J Allergy Clin Immunol* 79, 734–740.

Crema, A., del Tacca, M., Frigo, G.M. & Lecchini, S. (1968) Presence of a non-adrenergic inhibitory system in the human colon. *Gut* 9, 633–637.

Cutz, F., Levison, H. & Cooper, D.M. (1978) Ultrastructure of airways in children with asthma. *Histopathology* 2, 407–421.

Dahlen, S.E. (1983) Pulmonary effects of leukotrienes. *Acta Physiol Scand* 512 (Suppl), 1–51.

De Monchy, J.G.R., Kauffman, H.F., Venge, P. *et al.* (1985) Bronchoalveolar eosinophilia during allergen-induced late asthmatic reaction. *Am Rev Resp Dis* 131, 373–376.

Dunnill, M.S. (1960) The pathology of asthma, with special reference to changes in the bronchial mucosa. *J Clin Path* 13, 27–33.

Earle, B.V. (1953) Fatal bronchial asthma. A series of fifteen cases with a review of the literature. *Thorax* 8, 195–206.

Fabbri, L.M., Boschetto, P., Zocca, E. *et al.* (1987) Bronchoalveolar neutrophilia during late asthmatic reactions induced by toluene diisocyanate. *Am Rev Resp Dis* 136, 36–42.

Flint, K.C., Leung, K.B.P., Hudspith, B.N., Brostoff, J., Pearce, F.L. & Johnson, N. McI. (1985) Bronchoalveolar lavage mast cells in extrinsic asthma: a mechanism for the initiation of antigen specific bronchoconstriction. *Br Med J* 291, 923–926.

Gleich, G.J., Frigas, E., Filley, W.V. & Loegering, D.A. (1984) Eosinophils and bronchial inflammation. In Kay, A.B., Anslen, K.F., Lichtenstein, L.M. (eds), *Asthma Physiology, Immunopharmacology and Treatment,* pp. 195–210. Academic Press, London.

Glynn, A.A. & Michaels, L. (1960) Bronchial biopsy in chronic bronchitis and asthma. *Thorax* 15, 142–153.

Godard, P., Bousquet, J., Lebel, B. & Michel, F.B. (1987) Bronchoalveolar lavage in the asthmatic. *Bull Eur Physiopathol Resp* 23, 73–83.

Gonzalez, C., Diaz, P., Galleguillos, F., Ancic, P., Cromwell, O. & Kay, A.B. (1987) Allergen-induced recruitment of bronchoalveolar T helper (OKT4) and T suppressor (OKT8) cells in asthma: relative increases in OKT8 cells in single early-, as compared to late-phase responders. *Am Rev Resp Dis* 136, 600–604.

Hardy, C.C., Robinson, G., Tattersfield, A.E. & Holgate, S.T. (1984) The bronchoconstrictor effect of inhaled prostaglandin D_2 in normal and asthmatic man. *New Engl J Med* 311, 209–213.

Harris, H.W., Meneeley, G.R., Renzetti, A.D., Steele, J.D. & Wyatt, J.P. (1962) Definitions and classification of chronic bronchitis, asthma and pulmonary emphysema. *Am Rev Resp Dis* 85, 762–768.

Holgate, S.T., Hardy, C., Robinson, C., Agius, R.M. & Howarth, P.H. (1986) The mast cell as a primary effector cell in the pathogenesis of asthma. *J Allergy Clin Immunol* 77, 275–282.

Holgate, S.T., Beasley, R. & Twentyman, O.P. (1987) The pathogenesis and significance of bronchial hyperresponsiveness in airways disease. *Clin Sci* 73, 561–572.

Houston, J.C., de Navasquez, S. & Trounce, J.R. (1953) A clinical and pathological study of fatal cases of status asthmaticus. *Thorax* 8, 207–213.

Howarth, P.H., Durham, S.R., Kay, A.B. & Holgate, S.T. (1978) The relationship between mediator release and bronchial reactivity in allergic asthma. *J Allergy Clin Immunol* 80, 703–711.

Kneussl, M.P. & Richardson, J.B. (1978) α-Adrenergic receptors in human and canine tracheal and bronchial smooth muscle. *J Appl Physiol* 45, 307–311.

Lam, S., Le Riche, J., Phillips, D. & Chan-Yeung, M. (1987) Cellular and protein changes in bronchial lavage fluid after late asthmatic reaction in patients with red cedar asthma. *J Allergy Clin Immunol* 80, 44–50.

Lee, D.A., Winslow, N.R., Speight, A.N.P. & Hey, E.N. (1983) Prevalence and spectrum of asthma in childhood. *Br Med J* 286, 1256–1258.

Leyden, E.V. (1886) Ueber bronchial asthma. *Deutsch Militärarztl Zeitschr* 15, 51.

Metzger, W.J., Zavala, D., Richerson, H.B. *et al.* (1987) Local allergen challenge and bronchoalveolar lavage of allergic asthmatic lungs. *Am Rev Resp Dis* **135**, 433–440.

Nadel, J.A. (1977) Autonomic control of airway smooth muscle and airway secretions. *Am Rev Resp Dis* **115** (Suppl 2), 117–126.

Polak, J.M. & Bloom, S.R. (1982) Regulatory peptides in the respiratory tract of man and other animals. *Exp Lung Res* **3**, 313–328.

Polasa, R., Holgate, S.T. & Church, M.K. Adenosine as a pro-inflammatory mediator in asthma. *Pulmonary Pharmacology* (in press).

Salvato, G. (1968) Some histological changes in chronic bronchitis and asthma. *Thorax* **23**, 168–172.

Sheppard, N.M., Kuvian, S.S., Henzen-Logmans, S.C. *et al.* (1983) Neurone-specific enolase and S-100. New markers for delineating the innervation of the respiratory lining in man and other animals. *Thorax* **38**, 333–340.

Szentivanyi, A. (1968) The β-adrenergic theory of atopic abnormality in bronchial asthma. *J Allergy* **42**, 203–232.

Tattersfield, A.E., Holgate, S.T., Harvey, J.E. & Gribbin, H.R. (1982) Is asthma due to partial β-blockade of the airways. *Agents Actions* **13**, 265–271.

Weiss, S., Robb, G.P. & Ellis, L.B. (1932) The systemic effects of histamine in man. *Arch Int Med* **49**, 360–396.

Whitehead, W.E., Engel, B.T. & Shuster, M.M. (1980) Irritable bowel syndrome. Physiological and psychological differences between diarrhoea-predominant and constipation-predominant patients. *Dig Dis Sci* **25**, 404–413.

17 Food Intolerance and the Irritable Bowel Syndrome

J.O. Hunter

INTRODUCTION

In 1564 Queen Elizabeth I visited Cambridge and spent 5 days as the guest of the University. One of the highlights was an Act (or medical discussion) conducted in the University Church of Great St. Mary's with the Master of Caius College, Dr John Caius, on 'whether a simple diet was preferable to a varied one' (Venn, 1901). Over 400 years later modern gastroenterologists are again becoming aware of the importance of dietary factors in the production of functional gastrointestinal symptoms.

In the early years of the present century a number of American authors reported cases of diarrhoea and abdominal pain precipitated by eating specific foods (e.g. Duke, 1921, 1923; Rowe, 1928). However, this work was ignored by mainstream gastroenterologists in their studies of the irritable bowel syndrome (IBS), and it was not until 1982 that Alun Jones *et al.* described remission of symptoms in 14 out of 25 successive patients with IBS, 11 of which were subsequently objectively confirmed. Since then a number of studies of IBS have appeared, all of which confirm the presence of some patients with objective food intolerance (Bentley *et al.*, 1983; Farah *et al.*, 1985; Smith *et al.*, 1985). The incidence of patients with food intolerance in these reports varies from 6% (Farah *et al.*, 1985) to 60% (Alun Jones *et al.*, 1982). These differences are probably due to variations in patient selection, diet used and the method of challenge.

Patient selection

IBS is a diagnosis of exclusion and unfortunately, therefore, there is as yet no positive way of making the diagnosis. Ill-considered use of the term has lead to it becoming a convenient repository for any case with gastrointestinal symptoms for which the physician can find no cause, and it is commonplace nowadays to encounter patients with alleged IBS who in fact suffer from musculoskeletal problems (Ashby, 1977) or chronic hyperventilation (Lum, 1987).

The term IBS is probably best not used at all, because patients would be better labelled as 'unexplained diarrhoea' or 'unexplained abdominal pain and constipation'. Such terms might at least help to keep the supervising physician alert and thus avoid the mistaken supposition that a definite diagnosis has been reached.

The diagnosis of those patients with food-related gastrointestinal symptoms depends entirely on response to diet. Although a number of tests have been promoted as methods of making the diagnosis and identifying the foods concerned, there is none that has proved to be reliable (Sethi *et al.*, 1987). As it appears that food intolerance is not mediated by immunological mechanisms, skin tests and RAST tests are not relevant in the majority of cases, which therefore have to be identified on clinical criteria. Abdominal pain accompanied by diarrhoea and bloating is the symptom complex most likely to be associated with food intolerance, although a small number of patients may have predominant constipation. The symptoms which were encountered in a series of 122 patients studied at Addenbrooke's Hospital who were successfully treated are listed in Table 17.1.

Diet

The dietary regime used to identify patients with food intolerance has been explained in detail elsewhere (Workman *et al.*, 1984). In brief, there are three stages. In the first, which lasts for 2 weeks, patients are asked to keep to an 'exclusion diet' which avoids all those foods which are most likely to provoke symptoms, including most cereals and dairy products, citrus fruits, caffeine and yeast. Bulk laxatives may be necessary to maintain an adequate fibre intake. If there is no improvement after 2 weeks, the search for food intolerance is abandoned. The second stage begins when the patient finds that his symptoms have cleared. He then introduces the excluded foods one by one, eating each three to four times over a period of 2 days. This is usually long enough for the food to provoke a reaction, but it is necessary for the patient to keep a careful food diary, as some reactions are insidious and slow in their onset. Stage two is difficult for many patients because they suffer repeated unpleasant reactions and because at this stage initial enthusiasm for the diet has often waned. Stage three begins when all foods have been reintroduced and includes a dietary assessment for nutritional adequacy and ideally a double-blind challenge to confirm the food intolerance.

Challenge techniques

Many patients come to believe quite falsely that they suffer from food intolerances. This is particularly likely to occur when patients

Table 17.1. Symptoms suffered by 122 patients subsequently identifying food intolerances

Symptom	Incidence (%)
Abdominal pain	73
Diarrhoea	60
Tiredness	42
Headaches	38
Constipation	22.5
Abdominal distension	21.5
Fluid retention	20
Related conditions	
Migraine	11
Atopy	10

retrospectively blame unpleasant symptoms on a food they have previously eaten. The confirmation of food intolerance depends on the production of some unpleasant effect when the food concerned is given in a disguised form.

The development of classical immunology has influenced enormously the views of food intolerance that are held by patients and doctors alike. It is expected that most food reactions will follow the classical type I pattern, with a small amount of the food concerned (perhaps conveniently concealed in a capsule) giving rise to symptoms within a few hours of administration. In fact many patients can be shown to develop symptoms quite slowly after food administration. Indeed, it may take 2−4 days for some to react, especially if they are testing a food which had previously been avoided for several weeks (Fig. 17.1).

Although there are undoubtedly patients who develop symptoms as a result of a classical IgE-mediated reaction (Amlot *et al.*, 1987) and although Bentley *et al.* (1983) found that all their patients with IBS who had food intolerances were atopic, in our experience patients such as these are unusual (Hunter *et al.*, 1985). Gerrard (1979) has drawn attention to the phenomenon of 'delayed food allergy' in which symptoms develop slowly after administration of large amounts of the food in question, IgE concentrations are not raised and the incidence of atopic disorders is no greater than in the general population. We believe that many patients with functional gut disorders caused by food intolerance come into this group.

If patients with food intolerance are to be identified reliably the existence of such delayed reactions must be allowed for. Those patients with normal serum IgE concentrations must be tested with helpings of at least 100 g daily for at least 4 days. Much of the present confusion in the field of food intolerance is due to the failure of research workers to understand this phenomenon (Bentley *et al.*, 1983; Farah *et al.*, 1985). Challenges using small amounts of

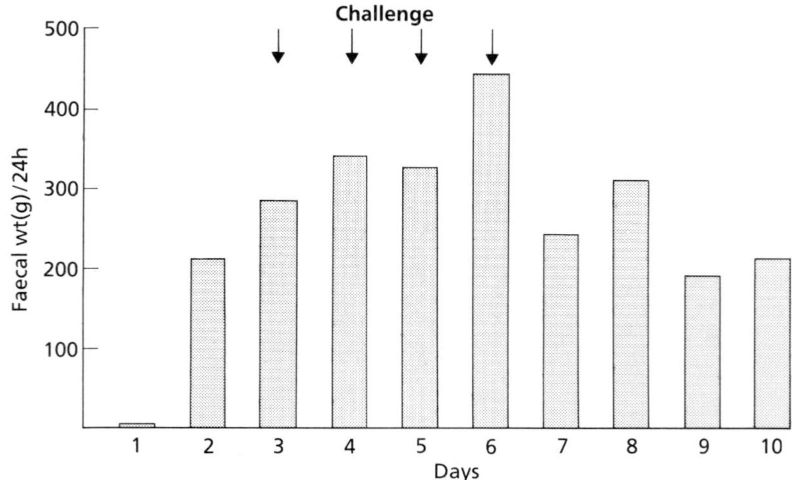

Fig. 17.1. Effect of a double-blind food challenge on faecal weight.

food will only reveal those patients with immunologically mediated disorders.

Long-term results

Patients with functional disorders of the gut are renowned for their frequent return visits to out-patients' clinics, because their symptoms persist and they need further reassurance, for both themselves and their medical advisers, that no serious pathology exists. One of the great advantages of the dietary approach is that patients achieve long-term control of their symptoms. Hunter *et al.* (1985) followed up through postal questionnaires a total of 193 patients who had been discharged from out-patients clinics between 2 and 39 months previously. 173 patients replied and of these 165 reported continuing benefit from their diets. Of those who had been discharged from the clinic between 22 and 39 months previously, 53 out of 61 were still well. Thus the initial effort expended in establishing a diet is usually well worthwhile.

Common food intolerances

The food intolerances detected by patients with functional gut disorders are usually very similar (Table 17.2). The great majority are intolerant of cereals and dairy products. Foods containing caffeine and yeast and citrus fruits are also very important but additives, preservatives and colourings are relatively infrequent. This pattern is virtually identical to that seen in other conditions including Crohn's disease (Alun Jones *et al.*, 1985), childhood

Table 17.2. Percentages of patients intolerant to particular foods

Food	Proportion of patients (%)	Food	Proportion of patients (%)	Food	Proportion of patients (%)
Cereals		Vegetables		Fruit	
Wheat	60	Onions	22	Citrus	24
Corn	44	Potatoes	20	Apples	12
Oats	34	Cabbage	19	Rhubarb	12
Rye	30	Sprouts	18	Banana	11
Barley	24	Peas	17	Strawberries	8
Rice	15	Carrots	15	Pineapple	8
		Lettuce	15	Pears	8
Dairy products		Leeks	15	Grapes	7
Milk	44	Broccoli	14	Melon	5
Cheese	39	Soya beans	13	Avocado pear	5
Butter	25	Spinach	13	Raspberries	4
Yogurt	24	Mushrooms	12		
		Parsnips	12	Miscellaneous	
Fish		Tomatoes	11	Coffee	33
White fish	10	Cauliflower	11	Eggs	26
Shell fish	10	Celery	11	Tea	25
Smoked fish	7	Green beans	10	Chocolate	22
		Cucumber	10	Nuts	22
Meat		Turnip/swede	10	Preservatives	20
Beef	16	Marrow	8	Yeast	12
Pork	14	Beetroot	8	Sugarbeet	12
Chicken	13	Peppers	6	Sugarcane	12
Lamb	11			Alcohol	12
Turkey	8			Tap water	10
				Saccharin	9
				Honey	2

migraine (Egger *et al.*, 1983) and hyperactivity (Egger *et al.*, 1985). The similarities suggest that there may be common pathogenetic mechanisms involved in all these conditions.

As many of these foods are staple items of Western diet, the discovery of food intolerances may provide social embarrassment. Unfortunately there is as yet no proven way of correcting food intolerances and it is therefore essential not to eat the foods if symptoms are to be prevented. This may lead to nutritional deficiencies. In our initial series of 182 patients treated by diet, 18 eventually had diets which were deficient in calcium and seven in iron. Three patients had diets deficient in vitamins A or D and two in vitamin C. One patient with a severely restricted diet was found to have an inadequate protein intake (Hunter *et al.*, 1985). It is essential that all patients undergoing dietary studies are supervised throughout by qualified dietitians. Unfortunately, many patients nowadays seek guidance on food intolerances from unqualified practitioners who use unproven techniques such as 'cytotoxic tests', 'hair analysis' and 'Vega machines'. These techniques have been shown to be unreliable (Sethi *et al.*, 1987) and it is nowadays all too common for such patients subsequently to present in outpatients' clinics following diets which are nutritionally inadequate.

FOOD ALLERGY—OR ENTEROMETABOLIC DISORDER?

It would be no exaggeration to state that the discovery of food intolerance has transformed the lives of many patients with functional disorders of the bowel. However, a dietary therapy is never ideal. Diets should be reserved for those conditions where no practical alternative exists (e.g. coeliac disease, IBS) or those such as Crohn's disease which are severe enough to justify the inconveniences involved. To establish a diet requires approximately 3–4 months of conscientious food testing with repeated unpleasant reactions when offending foods are encountered (Hunter *et al.*, 1985). It subsequently demands an iron self-discipline to eat only safe foods. Sadly but not surprisingly, a proportion of patients cannot cope with such a difficult task. It is therefore important to investigate the underlying mechanisms in the hope of identifying ways in which food intolerances might potentially be corrected and diet made unnecessary.

IMMUNOLOGICAL MECHANISMS

Although food reactions are referred to in common parlance as 'food allergy', it is clear that most patients with functional bowel disorders related to food do not have any immunological abnormality. Thus normal concentrations of IgE have been reported by several workers (Lessof *et al.*, 1980; Alun Jones *et al.*, 1982; Smith *et al.*, 1985). RAST tests are of little value in establishing the food intolerances present and the incidence of atopic disease in this group is no greater than that of the general population (10%) (Hunter *et al.*, 1985). Furthermore, the time course of the food reaction is slower than classical type I reactions and there is no increase in immune complexes, eosinophil count or plasma histamine after food challenge (Alun Jones *et al.*, 1982). Although it is still possible that there may be some unsuspected local immunological abnormality in the gut, it seems likely that the investigation of other recognized mechanisms of food intolerance may prove more rewarding.

Other mechanisms of food intolerance already recognized in general medicine are summarized in Table 17.3. It is possible that some or all of these may be involved in patients with functional gut disorders.

Chemicals in food
  Caffeine
  Ethanol
  Histamine
  Monosodium glutamate
Enzyme deficiencies
  Alactasia
  Monoamine oxidase inhibitors
Microbial breakdown of food residues
  Hepatic encephalopathy

Table 17.4. Pharmacologically active chemicals in food

Caffeine
Tyramine (cheese)
Histamine (cheese)
Phenylethylamine (chocolate)
Octopamine (citrus fruits)
Monosodium glutamate
Food additives, e.g. tartrazine

Chemicals in food

A list of chemicals which are commonly contained in food and which may produce idiosyncratic reactions is given in Table 17.4. Whilst many of these produce extraintestinal symptoms such as headache rather than affecting the gut, it is well known that many patients with functional gut disorders also suffer a wide range of symptoms including headache, fluid retention and tiredness (Whorwell *et al.*, 1986). Some chemicals may arise as a result of spoilage of the food (e.g. histamine in mackerel) in which case they may affect all subjects who eat them. Other chemicals (e.g. tyramine) clearly only affect a small proportion of the population in an adverse way (Hanington, 1983). These individuals are presumably different in some genetic way from their more resistant cousins and it is tempting to link such variation with differences in enzyme activity in the gut and liver.

Enzyme activity

Living organisms are exposed to a wide variety of dietary and environmental chemicals which they metabolize and excrete. Many of these chemicals are potentially toxic and the importance of the enzyme systems which deal with them should not be underestimated. Monoamine oxidase, for example, which is found in the liver, may be reduced in activity by the administration of drugs such as tranylcypromine and phenelzine. Subjects taking these drugs develop hypertension and headaches after eating foods which contain amines such as yeast, cheese and red wine. It has been shown that some subjects with dietary migraine have lower levels of monoamine oxidase in platelets than do control subjects (Sandler *et al.*, 1970; Glover *et al.*, 1977) and the levels of platelet phenol-sulphotransferase may also be reduced in this condition (Littlewood, 1982). However, the only common enzyme deficiency yet to be discovered in food intolerant diarrhoea is alactasia. It seems likely that other enzyme deficiencies will be discovered in this group.

Microbiological effects

One of the best known examples of food intolerance in clinical practice is the development of hepatic encephalopathy by cirrhotics whose dietary protein intake is excessive. The protein is broken down by the intestinal microflora with the production of chemicals, which are allowed to enter the systemic circulation because of the numerous collateral vessels which develop as a result of portal hypertension. Treatment with antibiotics such as neomycin is highly effective, and it is clear that the role of the bacterial flora in breaking down dietary protein to toxic amino compounds is of great importance.

The suggestion that toxic products might be derived by bacterial fermentation in the colon is far from new. Indeed, it was first proposed by Metchnikoff (1907). He suggested that constipation led to disease because of autointoxication by chemicals which were not eliminated sufficiently quickly. This theory is no longer accepted. However, it may be worth reconsidering a modern refinement of Metchnikoff's theory, proposing that constipation or the rate of transit itself is unimportant, but that specific foods may be metabolized to form toxic chemicals if damage occurs to the healthy flora of the colon.

There is some evidence in support of such a theory. Levitt (1976) reported a patient with alactasia who produced excessive volumes of rectal flatus. The gas was shown to comprise largely hydrogen and carbon dioxide. The hydrogen in particular could only have been produced by bacterial action, and dietary studies confirmed that it was a result of the bacterial fermentation of undigested milk sugar. It seems likely that subjects with normal levels of small intestinal lactase may also produce colonic gas in a similar fashion, for the same group showed hydrogen production in normal volunteers after ingestion of gluten-containing foods, but not after foods such as rice and sucrose which were completely absorbed in the small intestine (Anderson *et al.*, 1981). The presence of gluten in foods led to incomplete absorption of carbohydrate in the small intestine and its presentation to the caecal bacteria, which fermented it with the production of hydrogen.

It is now appreciated that as much as 40 g starch, 4 g fat, 14 g protein and 20 g fibre enter the caecum each day in normal individuals (Stephen, 1985). This provides a rich substrate for fermentation by the bacterial flora and it is known that short chain fatty acids and ammonia may be produced along with soluble waste products and hydrogen.

As hydrogen may easily be measured in the expired air, its release has provided a simple means of proving that a number of chemicals contained in food may reach the caecum in both normal subjects and patients with functional gut disorders. These include sugars such as sucrose (Bond *et al.*, 1981), fructose (Ravich *et al.*, 1983) and sorbitol (Hyams, 1983). Marked malabsorption of fructose and sorbitol but not of sucrose has recently been reported in functional bowel disorders. In seven out of 13 patients the fructose absorption capacities were below 15 g. Mixtures of 25 g fructose with 5 g sorbitol caused significant abdominal distress in these patients (Rasmussen & Gudmand-Hoyer, 1988). Starch malabsorption may be increased in normal subjects by the glucosidase inhibitor acarbose (BAY g 5421) and this also may lead to increases in stool weight and abdominal symptoms (Scheppach *et al.*, 1988).

Thus it is clear that sufficient substrate may enter the caecum from the small intestine to provide a basis for both bacterial fermentation and for the provocation of symptoms in susceptible individuals. Normal people, however, do not suffer symptoms as a result of bacterial fermentation. As food residues pass into the caecum in both subjects who develop symptoms and those who do not, it would seem likely that there must be differences in the bacterial flora of the two groups.

The microflora of the colon has not attracted the attention from gastroenterologists it truly deserves. This is partly because it is so complex; each gram of faeces may contain 10^{12} anaerobes and 10^6 aerobes and the assessment of changes in the faecal flora thus presents an enormous task. However, a number of observations have suggested that the colonic flora may be important in food intolerance. As we have seen, large quantities of food are required to produce reactions and the symptoms come on slowly. This time-scale is fully consistent with the hypothesis that food residues must be metabolized by colonic microorganisms to produce toxic chemicals. Furthermore, it is well known that functional diarrhoea may follow attacks of gastroenteritis or the administration of antibiotics (Alun Jones *et al.*, 1984). Both these events are known to be capable of inducing changes in the microflora (Van Der Waaij, 1983).

For these reasons we have made a particular study of the colonic

Table 17.5. Excretion of aerobic bacteria in faeces (viable bacteria/g dry weight faeces)

	n	Samples	Mean	Range
Patients	6	30	2.2×10^9	$2.9 \times 10^7 - 1.1 \times 10^{10}$
Controls	6	6	9.8×10^7	$3.9 \times 10^6 - 2.7 \times 10^8$

flora in food intolerance despite the technical difficulties involved. In preliminary experiments (Bayliss *et al.*, 1984) six patients were hospitalized and microbiological analysis of the faecal flora was carried out for 48 hours before and for up to 72 hours after challenge with wheat (five patients) or sugar (one patient). Similar studies were carried out in six age- and sex-matched controls. Higher numbers of aerobes were found in faecal samples from patients and in two patients, a 100-fold increase in the number of aerobes occurred during challenge (Table 17.5). There were noticeable changes in the predominant aerobic flora of four patients and anaerobic flora of three patients as judged by colony morphology and microscopy. Much lower numbers of bifidobacteria were isolated than expected (Croucher *et al.*, 1983).

Subsequently three detailed studies were carried out. A large scale blind study was performed in which levels of facultative bacteria, moisture content, pH and volatile fatty acids (VFAs) were determined on 103 stool samples from 101 patients (Bayliss *et al.*, 1986). These included a group of patients from a double-blind controlled hysterectomy study, which showed that treatment courses of antibiotics increased the vulnerability of patients to IBS (Alun Jones *et al.*, 1984), a group of patients with IBS presenting at medical outpatients before any dietary therapy, and a control group drawn from healthy hospital employees. Freshly passed stools were collected at home and transported under cool conditions to the laboratory within 5 hours.

The increased viable aerobic bacterial count discovered in the previous study was not confirmed as a significant difference in patients with IBS, as the counts were similar for both IBS and control categories (Table 17.6). However, assessment by questionnaires of the symptoms related to IBS in the hysterectomy patients showed that there was a significantly greater increase in symptom score in patients who had received postoperative courses of antibiotics than those receiving placebo or metronidazole prophylaxis ($P < 0.04$). Furthermore, stools from the former group of patients showed higher viable counts of aerobes. There was a significant correlation between the 3-month postoperative symptom score and aerobic bacterial count irrespective of drug treatment (Spearman's $\rho = 0.469$; $P = 0.009$).

Table 17.6. Faecal properties in food-related irritable bowel syndrome

	n	Log_{10} aerobic bacteria/g wet weight Mean	SE	Moisture content (%) Mean	SE	pH Mean	SE	n	Total VFA mol/g wet weight Mean	SE
All categories										
IBS	56	7.62	0.14	75.0	1.0	7.10	0.08	38	118	6
Control	35	7.47	0.16	72.2	1.0	7.10	0.08	34	112	5
'Naturally arising'										
IBS	38	7.65	0.14	74.4	1.2	7.09	0.10	26	125	7
Control	16	7.42	0.17	73.8	1.5	7.01	0.14	16	115	8
3 months' post-hysterectomy placebo only	5	7.04*	0.32							
Prophylaxis	10	6.80*	0.47							
Antibiotic treatment	18	7.82*	0.16							

* coefficient of contrast, $p = 0.018$

Escherichia and *Streptococcus* were the common genera in the stools. Other genera isolated were *Staphylococcus*, *Proteus*, *Klebsiella*, *Enterobacter* and *Micrococcus*. Genera other than *Escherichia* and *Streptococcus* were isolated from 17 out of 38 patients from the 'naturally arising' IBS group and four out of 16 controls, and from five out of 33 hysterectomy patients of whom four had a high symptom score. There was a decrease in the percentage of Gram-positive aerobic bacteria in the stools in the patient groups, although the decrease was not statistically significant.

These changes are similar to those observed by Balsari *et al.* (1982), who showed that with a group of IBS patients faecal coliforms were significantly reduced and that *Pseudomonas* and *Enterobacter* appeared in the stool. The changes in the flora of the patients studied supported the idea that in some patients with functional bowel disorders the state of the aerobic gut flora may be an indicator of the disease state, although further work is required to elucidate the full significance of these findings.

In a second study, two patients with food-related diarrhoea were admitted to hospital and the faecal microbial flora examined whilst they underwent double-blind food challenges (Wyatt *et al.*, 1988). Both patients displayed symptoms following challenge, and faecal output increased on the challenge diet although fibre content was kept constant. No significant diet-related differences in bacterial viable counts were seen in either patient (Table 17.7). The major short chain fatty acids present in both patients were acetic, propionic and *n*-butyric acids and in one patient the concentrations of all three increased markedly during the challenge diet. Both patients had a lower than usual ratio of anaerobic to aerobic bacteria in their faeces.

Table 17.7. Changes in faecal parameters in two patients during challenge with symptom-provoking food

Patient	Diet	Number of samples tested	(Mean (SE) $\log_{10}$ cfu/g*)		Anaerobe: aerobe ratio	Short chain fatty acids (mean (SE) µmol/g*)			Moisture content (mean (SE) %)
			Aerobes	Anaerobes**		Acetic	Propionic	*n*-Butyric	
P3	Normal	7	9.16	11.38	166:1	374	15.0	18.1	71.3
			(0.27)	(0.11)		(62.1)	(2.5)	(3.4)	(1.8)
			NS	NS		$P<0.05$	$P<0.05$	NS	NS
	Challenge	7	8.42	11.25	676:1	653[§]	30.9[§]	33.4[§]	74.7
			(0.15)	(0.05)		(75.6)	(4.5)	(6.8)	(2.6)
P7	Normal	10	8.7[†]	11.27[†]	372:1	289	42.2	69.2	79.6
			(0.08)	(0.06)		(33.6)	(5.8)	(15.9)	(0.71)
			NS	NS		NS	NS	NS	NS
	Challenge	10	8.98[††]	11.38[††]	251:1	292	38.5	89.2	80.1
			(0.13)	(0.04)		(21.3)	(4.6)	(13.9)	(0.71)

NS = no significant difference; values were compared by Student's t test; cfu = colony forming units.
* Dry weight; ** includes facultative anaerobes; [†] 9 samples tested; [††] 7 samples tested; [§] 6 samples tested.

A third patient suffering severe IBS related to food intolerances was also studied at various stages during her clinical course (Bradley *et al.*, 1986). Eight separate faecal samples were studied over an 18-month period. During this time the level of facultative organisms ranged from 72% to 0.7% and this seemed to correlate with her clinical state. The flora was very variable and there was an unusual incidence of *Clostridium* species.

These studies show that, although no pathogenic organisms are present in IBS, changes in some aspects of the gut flora may be associated with food-related diarrhoea, particularly the metabolic activity of the flora or the presence of increased numbers of aerobic species. These changes may move in different directions in different individuals and it is not certain whether they are the cause of the symptoms or just reflect other biological alterations. However, enough abnormalities have been discovered in the faecal flora of these patients to suggest that changes in the flora may indeed be the crucial factor in the pathogenesis of these conditions, even though the precise abnormality related to the bacteria concerned has still to be pinpointed.

Thus there is evidence to support all three features of the hypothesis that food intolerance is related to bacterial fermentation in the colon. Symptoms have been shown to be provoked by food, food residues can be shown to pass into the caecum and, although no specific pathogenic bacteria appear to be present, abnormalities of the bacterial flora have been demonstrated in these patients. Final confirmation of the hypothesis will depend on the identification of bacterial metabolites, produced in patients after ingestion of food provoking symptoms, but absent in normal controls eating the same diet.

Food allergy is a very inaccurate and inappropriate term to describe symptoms provoked by food in this manner. The symptoms are due to the metabolism of the food residues in the colon (and conceivably in other parts of the gut where bacterial contamination exists) and this process would be better described by the term 'enterometabolic disorder'. Whether other conditions apart from food-intolerant bowel disorders may also be considered as enterometabolic diseases remains a subject for speculation. Food intolerance is known to be important in migraine (Egger *et al.*, 1983) and asthma (Ogle & Bullock, 1977) and it is possible that such a mechanism is relevant in those conditions, for if it is possible for toxic metabolites to be produced which lead to spasm of smooth muscle in the gut, similar compounds might be produced which affect smooth muscle elsewhere in the body. Any such compounds would of course have to pass through the liver and this would be likely only to occur in subjects with reduced levels of certain hepatic enzymes. Thus the theory of enterometabolic disorders ties in well with evidence of enzyme deficiency previously described (Sandler 1970; Glover *et al.*, 1977; Littlewood *et al.*, 1982).

PRACTICAL APPROACH TO THE PATIENT WITH FUNCTIONAL GASTROINTESTINAL SYMPTOMS

Patients with gastrointestinal problems for which no pathological cause is apparent are extremely frequent in out-patients' clinics. It is important to avoid the patient becoming despondent about his prognosis or losing confidence in his physician. A practical strategy is therefore necessary to manage these patients as efficiently as possible.

It is necessary to do a number of investigations to exclude serious organic disease. In a young person a blood count, albumin concentration, acute phase proteins, ESR and stool culture should usually suffice. In all patients a sigmoidoscopy is mandatory, but a barium enema can usually be reserved for those whose symptoms have started over the age of 40.

Other conditions which it is important to exclude are musculoskeletal problems leading to abdominal pain, chronic hyperventilation and psychiatric disorders.

Musculoskeletal pains

It is very common for abdominal pain to arise in the muscles and joints of the spine and trunk and to radiate to the abdomen. Such pain is of course not accompanied by a change in bowel habit although it may temporarily become more severe after straining at stool. Musculoskeletal pain is present continuously for long periods of time, but tends to be relieved by resting in bed and is therefore less severe in the morning, getting worse as the day proceeds. It usually radiates to the back or to the leg and is made worse by physical exertion or by sitting for long periods in the same position, e.g. when driving a car. Unlike gut pain it is relieved by somatic analgesics.

Chronic hyperventilation

This condition has been described in detail elsewhere (Lum, 1987). Patients who hyperventilate characteristically suffer attacks of breathlessness associated with chest pain which radiates to the arms and with palpitations. They also frequently suffer gastrointestinal effects, including air swallowing, belching and gastric distension which may lead to upper abdominal discomfort. The distension and discomfort is characteristically relieved temporarily by belching and made worse by fizzy drinks. These patients all suffer from an underlying chronic anxiety state. Although some may improve with physiotherapy, which helps them to control their breathing correctly, more severe cases may require psychiatric support. Air swallowing may occur independently of hyperventilation and Calloway and Fonagy (1985) have stressed the importance of this in the production of functional gastrointestinal symptoms.

Psychiatric disorders

It is well known that both anxiety and depression may lead to gastrointestinal effects, but it is a mistake to search too vigorously for life-events which might be considered by the doctor, if not by the patient, as sufficient justification to produce abdominal pain. Most psychiatric problems are clinically clearly apparent. However, it should not be forgotten that both anxiety and depression may be secondary to the failures of previous medical advisors to deal effectively with the gastrointestinal symptoms of which the patient complains.

When these various disorders have been excluded, the next phase is to prescribe a bulk laxative such as ispaghula in adequate dosage for a period of 2–4 weeks. This not only ensures an adequate fibre intake but also may often improve symptoms such as diarrhoea and bloating. A high fibre diet may also be very helpful, but it is a mistake to equate fibre with wheat bran, as most patients with food intolerance have problems with wheat and will do badly on such a regime. Soya, oat and rice bran are all available and are superior to wheat bran for these patients.

In practice, the trial of ispaghula may be made whilst the results of the patient's investigations are awaited. If the patient's symptoms persist, the next step is to consider food intolerance. When the predominant symptom is bloating or diarrhoea there is little difficulty in deciding to try an exclusion diet. Constipation is less likely to respond and we prefer to measure the whole gut transit time (Fotherby & Hunter, 1987) to confirm genuine slow transit before embarking on an exclusion diet supplemented by adequate quantities of ispaghula.

Patients remain on the exclusion diet for 2 weeks. If at the end of that time they show no improvement they should be firmly advised that their problem is not related to food intolerance and to return to normal eating. Those patients who are better present few difficulties and continue with food reintroduction. Some patients claim a partial improvement. This may be due to a placebo effect, but may also be because the patients are intolerant of one or more of the foods which are permitted in the diet. In the latter case it is usually possible by examining their food diaries to decide which food is to blame. It is helpful to have the table of food frequencies (Table 17.2) available at this stage to provide a guide to likely offenders.

The process of food reintroduction may be slow and difficult but with application and care most patients can complete it successfully. A dietary analysis to ensure that the final diet is nutritionally adequate is essential and it is a good idea to perform one or more double-blind challenges if the patient will agree.

Those patients who do not improve on the exclusion diet should be reassessed and the possibility of hyperventilation reconsidered. It is my practice at this stage to inform these patients that their problem is probably related to stress, although this explanation is probably a cover for ignorance rather than the real truth. Be that as it may, it is often helpful then to advise management using the triple regime described by Truelove (1985).

CONCLUSIONS

The irritable bowel represents a testing challenge to gastroenterologists. It is not only the most common problem that they face but also the one which they treat most badly. Public dissatisfaction with the advice that they receive from their physicians is abundently apparent from the booming industry of alternative medicine and has spilled over even into the august columns of *The Times* (Anon., 1983). However, it is now possible to appreciate that IBS is a complex of many unrelated disorders, some of which have now been identified. Unfortunately they are not amenable to diagnosis through an endoscope and their separation and treatment is still only possible on clinical grounds. Nevertheless, this should not be beyond the wit of most gastroenterologists and prospects for sufferers from IBS continue to brighten.

Alun Jones, V., McLaughlan, P., Shorthouse, M., Workman, E. & Hunter J.O. (1982) Food intolerance: a major factor in the pathogenesis of irritable bowel syndrome. *Lancet* ii, 1115–1117.

Alun Jones, V., Wilson, A.J., Hunter, J.O. & Robinson, R.E. (1984) The aetiological role of antibiotic prophylaxis with hysterectomy in irritable bowel syndrome. *J Obstet Gynaecol* 5 (Suppl 1), S22–S23.

Alun Jones, V., Dickinson, R.J., Workman, E., Wilson, A.J., Freeman, A.H. & Hunter, J.O. (1985) Crohn's disease: maintenance of remission by diet. *Lancet* ii, 177–180.

Amlot, P.L., Kemeny, D.M., Zachary, C., Parkes, P. & Lessof, M.H. (1987) Oral allergy syndrome (OAS): symptoms of IgE-mediated hypersensitivity to foods. *Clin Allergy* 17, 33–42.

Anderson, I.H., Levine, A.S., Levitt, M.D. (1981) Incomplete absorption of the carbohydrate in all purpose wheat flour. *New Engl J Med* 304, 891–892.

Anon. (1983) Physician heal thyself. Editorial. *The Times*, 12th August, p. 9.

Ashby, E.C. (1977) Abdominal pain of spinal origin. Value of intercostal block. *Ann Roy Coll Surg Engl* 59, 242–246.

Balsari, A., Ceccarelli, A., Dubini, F., Fesce, E. & Poli, G. (1982) The faecal microbial population in the irritable bowel syndrome. *Microbiologica* 5, 185–194.

Bayliss, C.E., Houston, A.P., Alun Jones, V., Hishon, S. & Hunter J.O. (1984) Microbiological studies on food intolerance. *Proc Nutr Soc* 43, 16a.

Bayliss, C.E., Bradley, H.K., Alun Jones, V. & Hunter, J.O. (1986) Some aspects of colonic microbial activity in irritable bowel syndrome associated with food intolerance. *Ann Inst Super Sanita* 22, N3, 959–964.

Bentley, S.J., Pearson, D.J. & Rix, K.J.B. (1983) Food hypersensitivity in irritable bowel syndrome. *Lancet* ii, 295–297.

Bond, J.H., Currier, B.E., Buchwald, H. & Levitt, M.D. (1981) Colonic conservation of malabsorbed carbohydrate. *Gastroenterology* 78, 444–447.

Bradley, H.K., Wyatt, G.M., Bayliss, C.E. & Hunter, J.O. (1986) Instability in the faecal flora of a patient suffering from food-related irritable bowel syndrome. *J Med Microbiol* 22, 1–4.

Calloway, S.P. & Fonagy, P. (1985) Aerophagia and irritable bowel syndrome. *Lancet* ii, 1368.

Croucher, S.C., Houston, A.P., Bayliss, C.E. & Turner, R.J. (1983) Bacterial populations associated with different regions of the human colon wall. *Appl Env Microbiol* 45 (3), 1025–1033.

Duke, W.D. (1921) Food allergy as a cause of abdominal pain. *Arch Int Med* 28, 151–165.

Duke, W.D. (1923) Food allergy as a cause of illness. *JAMA* 81, 886–889.

Egger, J., Carter, C.M., Wilson, J., Turner, M.W. & Soothill, J.F. (1983) Is migraine food allergy? A double-blind controlled trial of oligoantigenic diet treatment. *Lancet* ii, 865–869.

Egger, J., Carter, C.M., Graham, P.J., Gurnley, D. & Soothill, J.F. (1985) Controlled trial of oligoantigenic therapy in the hyperkinetic syndrome. *Lancet* i, 540–545.

Farah, D.A., Calder, I., Benson, L. & Mackenzie, J.F. (1985) Specific food intolerance: its place as a cause of gastrointestinal symptoms. *Gut* 26, 164–168.

Fotherby, K.J. & Hunter, J.O. (1987) Idiopathic slow-transit constipation: whole gut transit times, measured by a new simplified method, are not shortened by opioid antagonists. *Aliment Pharmacol Therap* 1, 331–338.

Gerrard, J.W. (1979) The diagnosis of the food-allergic patient. In Pepys, J. & Edwards, A.M. (eds), *The Mast Cell: Its Role in Health and Disease*, pp. 416–421. Pitman Medical, Bath.

Glover, V., Sandler, M., Grant, E. *et al.* (1977) Transitory decrease in platelet monoamine oxidase activity during migraine attacks. *Lancet* i, 391–393.

Hanington, E. (1983) Migraine. In Lessof, M.H. (ed), *Clinical Reactions to Food*, pp. 155–180. Wiley, Chichester.

Hunter, J.O., Workman, E. & Alun Jones, V. (1985) The role of diet in the management of irritable bowel syndrome. In Gibson, P.R. & Jewell, D.P. (eds), *Topics in Gastroenterology 12*, pp. 305–313. Blackwell Scientific Publications, London.

Hyams, J.S. (1983) Sorbitol intolerance: an unappreciated cause of functional gastrointestinal complaints. *Gastroenterology* 84, 30–33.

Lessof, M.H., Wraight, D.G., Merrett, T.G., Merrett, J. & Buisteret, P.D. (1980) Food allergy and intolerance in 100 patients. *Q J Med* 195, 259–271.

Levitt, M.D. (1976) Studies of a flatulent patient. *New Engl J Med* 295, 260–262.

Littlewood, J. (1982) Platelet phenosulphotransferase deficiency in dietary migraine. *Lancet* i, 983–986.

Lum, L.C. (1987) Hyperventilation syndrome in medicine and psychiatry: a review. *J Roy Soc Med* 80, 229–231.

Metchnikoff, E. (1907) *The Prolongation of Life*. Heinemann, London.

Ogle, K.A. & Bullock, J.D. (1977) Children with allergic rhinitis and/or bronchial asthma treated with elimination diet. *Ann Allergy* 39, 8.

Rasmussen, J.J. & Gudmand-Hoyer, R.T. (1988) Functional bowel disease: malabsorption and abdominal distress after ingestion of fructose, sorbitol and fructose-sorbitol mixtures. *Gastroenterology* 95 (3), 694–700.

Ravich, W.J., Bayless, T.M. & Thomas, M. (1983) Fructose: incomplete intestinal absorption in humans. *Gastroenterology* 84, 26–29.

Rowe, A.H. (1928) Food allergy: its manifestations, diagnosis and treatment. *JAMA* 91, 1623–1631.

Sandler, M., Youdim, M.B.H., Southgate, J. & Hanington, E. (1970) The role of tyramine in migraine: some possible biochemical mechanisms. In Cochrane, A.L. (ed), *Background to Migraine. 3rd Migraine Symposium*, pp. 103–112. Heinemann Medical, London.

Scheppach, W., Fabian, C., Ahrens, F., Spengler, M. & Kasper, H. (1988) Effect of starch malabsorption on colonic function and metabolism in humans. *Gastroenterology* 95, 1549–55.

Sethi, T.J., Kemeny, D.M., Tobin, S., Lessof, M.H., Lambourn, E. & Bradley A. (1987) How reliable are commercial allergy tests? *Lancet* i, 92–94.

Smith, M.A., Youngs, G.R. & Finn, R. (1985) Food intolerance, atopy and irritable bowel syndrome. *Lancet* ii, 1064.

Stephen, A.M. (1985) Effect of food on the intestinal microflora. In Hunter, J.O. & Alun Jones, V. (eds), *Food and the Gut*, pp. 57–77. Baillière Tindall, Eastbourne.

Truelove, S.C. (1985) Treatment. In Jewell, D.P. & Gibson, P.R. (eds), *Topics in Gastroenterology 12*, pp. 289–304. BSP, London.

Van der Waaij, D. (1983) *Antibiotic Choice: the Importance of Colonisation Resistance*. Research Studies Press, Chichester.

Venn, J. (1901) *Caius College*. Cambridge University Press, Cambridge.

Whorwell, P.J., McCallum, M., Creed, F.H. & Roberts, C.T. (1986) Non-colonic features of irritable bowel syndrome. *Gut* 27, 37–40.

Workman, E., Hunter, J.O. & Alun Jones, V. (1984) *The Allergy Diet*. Dunitz, London.

Wyatt, G.M., Bayliss, C.E., Lakey, A.F., Bradley, H.K., Hunter, J.O. & Alun Jones, V. (1988) The faecal flora of two patients with food-related irritable bowel syndrome during challenge with symptom-provoking foods. *J Med Microbiol* 26, 295–299.